CRAFTS   ABLED

<u>FOR ALL AGES</u>

Crafts for the Very Disabled And Handicapped

By

JANE G. KAY

Former Activities Director, Human Services Department
Central Piedmont Community College
Charlotte, North Carolina

Volunteer Arts and Crafts Coordinator
Nursecare Nursing Center
Charlotte, North Carolina

Psychometrist, Educational Improvement Project
Tulane University
New Orleans, Louisiana

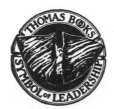

CHARLES C THOMAS · PUBLISHER
Springfield · Illinois · U.S.A.

Published and Distributed Throughout the World by
CHARLES C THOMAS • PUBLISHER
Bannerstone House
301-327 East Lawrence Avenue, Springfield, Illinois, U.S.A.

© 1977, by CHARLES C THOMAS • PUBLISHER
ISBN 0-398-03661-6
Library of Congress Catalog Card Number: 77-1914

Library of Congress Cataloging in Publication Data

Kay, Jane G.
  Crafts for the very disabled and handicapped.

  Bibliography: p.
  1. Handicraft. 2. Handicapped—Recreation.
I. Title.
TT157.K38   745.5   77-1914
ISBN 0-398-03661-6

Printed in the United States of America
C-11

TO

JENNIFER AND JONATHAN

Give to the world the best that you have,
and the best will come back to you.

Preface

THE EXTREMELY DISABLED or handicapped person (who may or may not be institutionalized) needs to feel useful with some degree of the integrity and self-esteem our society places upon independence. This book is not a scientific or a theoretical production; but rather, it is an effort to present a compilation of material based upon many real-life experiences with disabled and handicapped people and the development of craft therapy at its simplest level. This book differs from other craft books in that not only are the projects intended to hold the interest of adults, but also the need of professional people and volunteers alike to have explicit instructions with detailed patterns and diagrams is taken into account.

The crafts in this book are simple enough for the very disabled and handicapped yet not belittling to geriatric patients. Although the crafts I suggest are suitable for many ages, I am mainly concerned with nursing home residents. Those with whom I tried out the projects ranged from the physically able but very senile to the extremely disabled but mentally alert. So in this book lies a collection of carefully planned projects for the young and old. The projects are not hazardous for feeble minds and even enable shaking hands to use common tools and materials in an essential type of recreation in modern day society.

I hope that the projects described herein will suggest new means of coping with the many idle hours that beset the extremely disabled and handicapped, whether their problems be physical, social, or emotional.

JANE G. KAY

Acknowledgments

IT IS A PLEASURE to acknowledge the many friends who have offered their help and have been so gracious as to share their ideas and enthusiasm.

My wholehearted thanks to Betty Droescher, Arthur Wallace, Beth Capper, Shirley Eaker, and Harry Swimmer.

A special message of appreciation to Michael Kay, my husband and friend, who has given much encouragement and valuable help.

And most of all I thank the residents of Nursecare, a group of people who share a wisdom and understanding of life known only to the infirm among us.

J.G.K.

Contents

CRAFTS FOR THE VERY DISABLED AND HANDICAPPED

CHAPTER ONE

The Disabled and Handicapped

IT IS COMMON KNOWLEDGE that major technological and medical advances are helping to save lives today of those who not long ago would have died. Of course, it is hoped that scientific discoveries will eventually lead to the prevention or cure of all disease and illness commonly known as physical disability. In the meantime, however, fulfilling activities must be provided for the lives saved by today's degree of technology.

Today there is improved health care available to the poor and those in outlying areas. The infant mortality rate is declining along with the birth rate. Research is bringing cancer, heart, and vascular diseases under more control. The net result is a growth in not only the sixty-five-and-over age-group but also the number of the enfeebled aged who once would have died. Likewise, premature infants, children, and adults ill with acute infections or the injuries of accidents also live. But they live with gross alterations in physique and with severe impairments in physiological functioning.

Although medicine has made phenomenal advancements, such as those against polio and against blindness caused by an untreated mother's syphilis, realistically, there is little hope that disability and illness will disappear. Cures must be found for impaired vision of juvenile diabetes, arthritis, cerebral palsy, spina bifida, and paralysis from stroke among others. Illness and disability are not disappearing. Rather, the number of extremely disabled people throughout the world is escalating.

Everyone has the right to medical care and the improvements in preventive medicine, but the poor and aged are not truly benefitting from better medical care. Most medical students still head to make their livings in urban centers. And far too many patients hear that they are just growing old from somatic complaints rather than getting exhaustive physical examinations that might prevent later disasters and crippling diseases. This phenomenon is understandable; until recently, there were few corrections available for discovered dysfunctions. But today, preventive geriatrics should be encouraged because disabling diseases can be controlled, or at the very least, they are more manageable when discovered early.

Thus it appears that physical disability is often the price of saving lives. What is a physical disability as distinct from a handicap? The term disability denotes a medical-physical defect or impairment. Intrinsically, disability refers to an inability to meet certain standards of physical efficiency. It differs from disease in that it does not refer to the fundamental biological needs of life. Physical disability might be considered to be the antithesis of capability or physical fitness, while that of illness is health.

The term handicap used to be a colloquialism for the crippled or physically unfit. However, today handicap refers to an impairment in a particular kind of social and psychological behavior. Inherent in this distinction is the fact that handicaps do not always coincide with a disability. It might be useful to look at an example: Diabetes is an illness; childhood blindness resulting from this illness is a disability; problems of adjustment in coping with the blindness is a handicap. Thus it becomes useful to distinguish between physical limitations and the resultant psychological and social impairments for understanding why people with the same physical disabilities may behave differently.

It should be noted that physical disabilities are relative to the culture in which they occur. For example, in our society a bilateral hand amputee would be disabled. However, in China's traditional culture, when a man was approaching the pinnacle of success, he closed his hands into fists and allowed his finger nails to grow through the palms to the other side. Although he lost the use of his hands, he gained recognition and prestige by showing he had servants to care for him and did not have to resort to common labor. In light of this, it can be said that a disability exists only when a person lacks the means for behavior that his culture deems important. While some frequent debilitating diseases are heart and vascular ailments, cardiovascular accidents, malignant diseases, impairments in the locomotor system, mental disturbances, and endocrine disorders, it is not feasible to discuss all physical disabilities. Amputations are obvious, while brain tumors are hidden. Let it suffice to say that there is a vast number of disabilities running the gamut of human life.

Although one might attempt to define disability, all delineations are complicated by social judgments. Social prejudice can and does effect behavior. Although serious attempts are made to understand disabilities and handicaps, there is still derisive contempt for cripples and unfair state laws against epileptics. It is simply a fact that although some physical disabilities are socially handicapping only, they are still perceived by the majority as undesirable. Examples of these social prejudices are those based on physical attributes such as race, sex, and age. Fair or not, these social stereotypes determine how a person is expected to behave and what he will be permitted to do. Thus, socially imposed handicaps on people with atypical physiques are important to the overall understanding of physical disability. A person raised to think of himself as a "cripple" (a term with so many negative connotations) will behave as he thinks society expects. An elderly person will behave likewise when he hears such negative colloquialisms as "over the hill" and "out to pasture."

It is understandable that physical defects and social handicaps place individuals under particular stress. However, except in cases which are almost totally disabling, the significance of these impairments in the development of emotional handicaps depends primarily upon the way the individual evaluates and adjusts to his unusual or changed life situation. In many cases, the physical disability is an excuse for, and not the cause of, psychological maladjustment. The main problems which occur are resignation and feelings of inferiority, self-pity, fear, and hostility. In effect, the individual listens to society and devaluates himself. It is important to note again that the attitude toward the disability seems to be the salient variable in emotional adjustment. Hence, there is the potential for good adjustment with a severe physical disability and widespread emotional handicaps with only slight physical defects.

Although disability, social handicap, and emotional handicap have been explained independently and separately from each other, combinations of handicaps are the rule rather than the exception. Of course, impairments may be small. However, they are often chronic. Too often, the chronically ill patient becomes isolated and ignored. No one wants to spend time with him because he is depressing, exhausting, insoluble, and irreversible. A chain reaction occurs. The lessened social interaction of the individual leads to loneliness and isolation reducing at the same time his resources for coping with his problems. The ensuing stress in turn contributes to illness. The person begins to play a role of being sick. Is there a better cure for pain or a better balm for emotional ills than feeling useful or playing a truly meaningful role in society? But who will help a grossly impaired person with multiple disabilities and handicaps who lives only because modern medical miracles saved him at so high a cost?

CHAPTER TWO

Craft Therapy

TRADITION AND SOCIAL prejudice has relegated the victims of stroke, senility, psychoses, mental retardation, cerebral palsy, cancer, and other extremely debilitating diseases to an almost subhuman status. The disabled seem to be no longer entitled to be treated as relatives, friends, and human beings. They are frequently banished to convalescent and nursing homes, where someone else assumes their care. Clearly attitudes must be changed. And changes are coming, both within the medical profession and without.

Large numbers of professionals are devoting their lives to the practice of rehabilitation via art therapy and/or occupational therapy. Through new methods of rehabilitation, the individual with physical or emotional impairments is given the opportunity for improved independence and personal care. He is taught to discover latent potentialities. At the very least, rehabilitation techniques strive to arrest any further decline in functional capacity.

One method of helping patients with adjustment problems is art therapy. The psychologist or social worker trained to work with the emotionally disturbed analyzes art work done by the patient. This method of therapy typifies the flexibility and perceptiveness necessary for dealing with emotional handicaps, as the disturbed often cannot express or indeed even understand their own problems, fears, and frustrations. If they cannot communicate to the therapist, the therapist may learn to understand them through the hidden messages and symbols in their art. The artwork is seen as a mural of the mind; therefore the artwork is not an end in itself but rather is a tool of rehabilitation. Needless to say, the art therapist is highly skilled and trained in dealing with behavior disorders.

Another method of rehabilitation is occupational therapy. Although occupational therapy has often been identified exclusively with handicrafts, its main purpose is to ensure improvements of independence in the activities of daily living. The medical and nursing team, along with the physical therapists, helps the patient improve his functional capacity. The occupational therapist helps him perform independently. The occupational therapist teaches the patient everything from getting up in the morning to going to bed at night, including washing, shaving, dressing, eating, reading, leisure pursuits, and a host of other activities. Like the art therapist, the occupational therapist is highly skilled and trained to accomplish basic aims. The occupational therapist must know how to assess functional capacities and limitations, how to improve function with the patient's cooperation, and how to heighten social competence.

The occupational therapist does not want to be associated only with handicrafts. Thus the training books mention crafts as a means of coping with leisure time but do not teach craft techniques for impaired people. On the other hand, the philosophy of the creative artist does not include pattern books with detailed instructions and diagrams. Then too, these therapists are highly trained to know the pathological bases of various impairments. They know which patients are good candidates for rehabilitation and which patients are not. Too often the grossly impaired individuals are ignored for the more satisfying job of seeing one's skilled training come to fruition in the more total rehabilitation of lesser disabled patients. The extremely disabled and handicapped person is left with nothing to do, nothing to talk about, nothing to think about, and nothing to live for.

Great numbers of the disabled and handicapped cannot truly hope to be returned to society yet need "craft therapy." So it is that the object of rehabilitation for these long-term patients with no chance of recovery is remotivation in terms of resocialization, activities, and a sense of worth. Of course, the hope is always for improvement, but the realistic goal is for mere diversional activities to give the patient some interest outside himself and some goal to pursue that is within his ability to function. This diversional activity helps to deal with unbearable boredom. The crafts in this book are designed for such activity.

One of the worst problems faced by the therapist is the task of motivating the patients. Perhaps when a patient experiences individual creative success, he will venture toward the more competitive environment of a small group. There, if even a passive participant of the group, he enters into the resocialization process. He moves toward some degree of independent action within the framework of the social structure of life in his institution. And eventually he may even pursue the traditional creative arts that allow self-expression.

Ideally, the craft therapist should know the individual case history of each patient. Like the occupational therapist, he should be familiar with medical and psychological terminology. He should be able to know just what each patient can and cannot do. He should know each patient's interests. Did this person have any special interests or hobbies before the disability? Is the patient willing to try anything new? Is he an optimist or a pessimist? Is he feeling sorry for himself; does he have a chip on his shoulder?

Since obviously there are as many personalities as there are people, it would be best for a therapist to know individual traits and abilities. Unfortunately, the craft therapist is often only a part-time activities' director or volunteer. If a therapist goes into the activities room with a shortage of volunteers and twenty-five apprehensive, enfeebled patients waiting to feel useful to themselves and society, what should he do? He can hardly tat with one and oil paint with another; throw clay pots and do woodwork, needlepoint and macramé. Projects with general appeal and a low level of difficulty are needed. The problem is that simple projects are often looked upon as child's play by adults and, to quote an elderly patient whose therapist helped with a detailed project, "You do it for us and then tell us how good we are—nonsense!"

The importance of a feeling of self-worth cannot be stressed enough. While children can do almost any craft project, adults cannot. Even the most enfeebled geriatric patient has a lifetime of experience that tells him right away when some project is simple activity as distinct from purposeful activity. Meaningful activity is associated with a satisfactory level of self-esteem, positive feelings about life, and higher morale. Most very disabled and handicapped patients have given up. With good results on the simple projects presented in the following chapters, these patients will be ready to advance as their self-confidence builds.

Remember that the elderly patient does not learn as quickly or retain new information as long as a child. Consequently, longer periods of time are needed to accomplish seemingly simple tasks. And the tasks themselves should be kept simple to minimize frustration and stress. Incentives are a must. The older patient grew up believing that work was good and idleness was sinful. Thus, the projects he attempts must still be deemed valuable by him. The therapist is not apt to pull the wool over anybody's eyes with simple busywork.

Although the craft projects in this book are limited to a low level of difficulty, they are truly useful to the patients and to society. The projects are separated by chapter as to their particular uses. There are ten projects in each chapter. Of course, some of the uses are multiple. But all in all, the arrangement of the book is intended to provide a year's projects (if taken weekly). Some of the crafts are more suitable for a holiday season while others, such as Strawberries, are good summer projects.

The projects just to enjoy are meant for the patients themselves. Although all projects should be geared to having a use in society, many patients do not want to part with their creations. At the very least, the first or best one of a particular project is usually carried back to the patient's room. And who does not derive pleasure from his own accomplishments? Sometimes a participant in group crafts will say he does not like or want his project. The therapist need not insist. Perhaps another patient would like it. Or it might be displayed on a shelf in the activities room. Its owner will still feel good about his accomplishment. A therapist must remember never to be overly complimentary. The patient knows how well he has done. When he is ready to accept his achievements, he will.

Before this author ever walked into an activities room to present a craft program, staff members warned that the participants would be extremely disabled and handicapped. At the first session an assortment of people were present: an arthritic patient with Parkinson's disease, a manic depressive, several chronic brain-disordered patients, a paralyzed stroke victim, a young spina bifida victim, a terminal cancer patient, a retarded arsonist released from a hospital for the criminally insane, and a cruelly disfigured catatonic just barely functioning after thirty-five years in the state mental hospital. These were the ambulatory patients who were motivated enough to even come to a crafts session! There were countless others either not motivated to ever leave their rooms or nonambulatory. Then, too, there were patients in intensive and skilled care who simply were not able to participate in even a bedside crafts program. It was for this latter group that projects were made by the more able participants.

Families play a large role in the lives of patients. They are a link to the outside world. Children want to show their accomplishments for approval. Parents and grandparents want some token to give to visitors, as they often do not have the means to shop for gifts.

Patients often produce item after item for family members who never come to visit. The greatest sense of self-esteem for these patients seems to come from projects that are given to agencies. Most cities have volunteer bureaus which are hungry for any type of handicraft. They will distribute the projects to appropriate recipients and will send a nice letter of appreciation to show to the patients. The Veterans Administration, children's hospitals, schools, Head Start, and church bazaars are only a few of the agencies that will make good use of the projects. Police and fire departments may be asked what they can use. Bookmarks can be given to libraries. All projects should be given with a note about how and why they were made. There should be no embarrassment about the quality of workmanship or about asking for a letter of appreciation in return for the projects.

The typical institution has a boutique or gift shop. For so long, personal worth has been measured by financial success. This idea dies hard. Some patients only feel useful with some degree of the integrity and esteem our society places upon independence when their craft projects are sold. There is no question that seeing one's own work come to fruition is gratifying. A small display case in the lobby or hall of any institution might be set up. Each resident could participate by contributing know-how, arts and crafts items, or work time. There could be either profit sharing or simply selling the items on consignment. At the nursing home where the author works, all the patients decided to pool the income to buy a kiln. No doubt it will take a long time, but it is a common goal.

The crafts presented in the following chapters have been rated as to level of difficulty. One asterisk denotes an extremely simple and unchallenging project; two asterisks mark a more difficult project, and so on up to five. (Projects are usually marked with two groups of asterisks to show the range of difficulty.) This is a subjective value judgment on the part of the author. Just as two people with the same physical disability can have radically different behavior, they also have a different performance of tasks depending upon their interests and motivations.

A project with one asterisk might be very repetitive and excellent therapy for a senile patient, or it might be simple enough for a blind patient. Although a project such as Paper Flowers is suitable for the senile and blind, it might also appeal to more able or alert patients for a shorter period of time.

Each of the projects that has five asterisks necessitates a higher level of eye-hand coordination or more attention to detail. However, there is an exception to every rule. When the therapist works bedside in a one-to-one relationship, even the very enfeebled can accomplish most of the projects in this book.

Actually, the rating system is relative at best, as all the projects were designed for an exceptionally low level of ability. It is simply that some projects are better for some impairments, while other projects are better for others. For example, the bold outlines of the patterns for Coasters make them easy to see for the visually impaired, and since any coloring out of lines is cut away from the pattern, it is a good project for hands that shake. Likewise, since tremor often improves or disappears with purposeful function, Potato Print Cards are especially good for parkinsonians. On the other hand, paints are not good for shaking hands unless you have very understanding aides, who do not mind doing extra bathings of bodies and washings of clothes. If the instructions are read like recipes, and a physical therapist is used when possible the best combinations of disorders and crafts will soon be learned.

The crafts presented in this book can almost all be completed in one session of approximately an hour. The craft therapist should be patient: The patients have nothing but time. Help and interference on a project may produce more finished products per hour but they will not help the patient feel he did it himself. There is an almost overwhelming urge to help disabled and handicapped people, especially when they say "I cannot do it!" The therapist should not give in too easily to negative responses. While the therapist should not badger a patient, some degree of participation should be insisted upon. He should put a crayon in the patient's hand and say "Color this area with this red crayon." Then, the therapist should compliment the patient honestly and encourage him with such expressions as "Why, Mr. Richardson, you had me buffaloed all these weeks . . . for shame!" The response will probably be a smile. If nothing else works, let the patient observe a project while talking nonchalantly about other things. He might be intrigued enough to try it next time.

The projects are of short duration to help cope with short attention spans. The more traditionally creative arts take more than one sitting. Often as the patient becomes older, his mind forgets from day to day, so these projects can almost all be completed in one session. Each patient prefers to do his own project. While sometimes patients would work in teams, most did not like assembly-line crafts. Each wants his project to be his own.

The importance of having samples of each project to show at the beginning of each craft session cannot be stressed enough. If professionals and volunteers cannot visualize a handicraft without a drawing, how can the extremely disabled and handicapped be expected to do so? In fact, one should always try to bring several finished items of each project to display, for example, Dresser Scarves with a variety of patterns or Easter Eggs with simple and detailed designs.

Bringing finished samples leads to a discussion of preparation ahead of time. A good deal of preparation ahead of time makes for foolproof craft projects. Of course, a true artist would argue vehemently with this point of view, because it takes away from creativity and self-expression. But many of these enfeebled people do not have the incentive to get out of bed. They are a long way from creative self-expression. With patience, understanding, and successful experiences on simple projects, the patient may later develop creativity. The therapist should always be on the lookout for the potential artist and encourage his self-expression whenever possible. In the meantime, it is necessary to provide patterns for those who otherwise would do nothing.

The preparation done at home for the teaching of crafts is often grueling. But if the therapist pulls threads and draws patterns on a dresser scarf while a patient watches, and if the patient is then told to color it, he will feel that he is not doing much. But if the patient comes into a room and the scarves are ready to color, he will not think too much about how they got there. The project becomes his. Any preparation ahead of time is well worth the effort.

Craft supplies, of course, should be safe and nontoxic. Common sense should be used in choosing them: Senile patients often put almost anything into their mouths, and manic depressives ought not to have scissors in their rooms. There are a number of economical ways of acquiring craft supplies, short of stealing. Seeds, meat trays, produce baskets, cans, medicine cups, etc. can be saved. The Yellow Pages will have a list of any local factories where boxes, fabric, buttons, trim, cans, colored paper, etc. can be found. Nature may be used as a veritable storehouse of supplies if one keeps one's eyes open.

Rapport and trust are essential in order to gain cooperation. This, more than anything else, often tests the therapist's or volunteer's ability to present a successful program of craft activities. In meeting the disabled, it is often hard to get past the handicap stigma. One handicapped person expressed it well in saying that there seem to be eyes everywhere—eyes that slide away in revulsion or dislike, eyes filled with pity (a crippler in itself), eyes that go blank, and eyes that stare. If the therapist enjoys encounters with disabled people the patients know. Nonverbal behavior gives one away. If one is constrained, nervous, or stilted, the patients will be embarrassed.

The best advice that can be given is to "be honest and be yourself." The extremely disabled and handicapped, especially the geriatric patient, is coping with the basics of life. He knows his situation; the therapist knows his situation. Reality must not be denied, and yet one must continue in spite of it. Since reality is hard enough to cope with, the patient should not be asked to deal with make-believe too. Celebrate the life existing today. It will not help to live in the future ("What's it worth?") or to dwell in the past ("He was such an active, vital person before this impairment"). Handicapped people can learn to cope with their affliction in time, but the embarrassment the impairment causes others is almost unbearable. Help should not be given unless asked for; one should not talk in hushed, mournful tones. Illness is a part of the full circle of life, as is death. Research today points to the needs of all people, even the terminally ill, for honesty.

These people who have lived a full circle of life have many intangibles to give. They can be fun and interesting to talk to, and they are very grateful for anything, that is done for them. They seem to have a wisdom and understanding of life that would be well worthwhile to learn. Of course, some patients are moody at times or difficult to help. Some are withdrawn and often try the therapist's patience in attempting to motivate them. The therapist should try to realize they are ill and infirm. While the therapist helps the patient do something useful and feel worthwhile, the patient will be helping the therapist do something useful and feel worthwhile. It is only a value judgment to say who does the best job!

If at all possible, a reality orientation program should be introduced. Patients in nursing homes often become confused and disoriented. If there is not an active reality orientation program, it would help for the therapist to always wear a name tag with letters large enough to be seen. The author's tag says "Hello. My Name is Janie Kay. What's Yours?" The author always had the patients in group crafts also wear name tags. All staff members should preface sentences with names when addressing individuals. The therapist should become a regular part of the patients' lives and stop by each room for a smile and a "hello" even when he cannot provide a daily bedside craft for everyone. At least the therapist will provide some continuity.

Dr. Robert Butler in *Why Survive?* expressed not only the problems of the aged but also those of all the infirm among us:

After one has lived a life of meaning, death may lose much of its terror. For what we fear most is not really death but a meaningless and absurd life. I believe most human beings can accept the basic fairness of each generation's taking its turn on the face of the planet if they are not cheated out of the full measure of their own turn . . . we still have the possibility of making life a work of art.

CHAPTER THREE

Craft Projects Just to Enjoy

BEADS

Level of difficulty: *—*****

MATERIALS: Salt, flour, vegetable colorings, darning needle, cord such as No. 30 crochet cotton, round toothpicks, wax paper, dried seeds and old broken strands of beads, nail polish.

APPLICATIONS: By varying the colors and shapes, you can make many attractive strings. By varying the lengths of the strings, you can make bracelets, necklaces, or belts. Some people with fairly nimble fingers may want to tie a small knot between each bead or seed to make a more attractive strand.

PREPARATION BEFORE CRAFT SESSION: Mix two thirds of a cup of salt, a cup of flour, one third of a cup of water, and two or three drops of vegetable coloring. This will form a heavy dough. Make the dough in a variety of colors. To prepare the seeds for stringing, soak the seeds in water for a day or two. Then pierce a hole with a needle in each seed. You may want to paint some of the seeds with nail polish.

CRAFT SESSION: Have each person roll a small amount of the dough between the palms of his hands to shape it. Make a hole with a toothpick in the center of each bead as soon as it is finished. Lay the beads on wax paper to dry. Some people might only be able to shape beads, while others may prefer to punch holes. Make an assembly line. Look at the illustrations for stringing the beads and seeds.

SALT BEADS

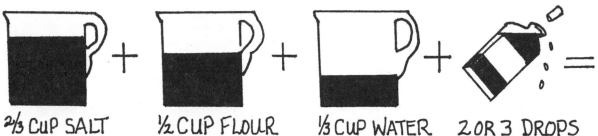

²⁄₃ CUP SALT + ½ CUP FLOUR + ⅓ CUP WATER + 2 OR 3 DROPS VEGETABLE COLORING.

MIX IN A SMALL BOWL.
THIS IS MODELING DOUGH.

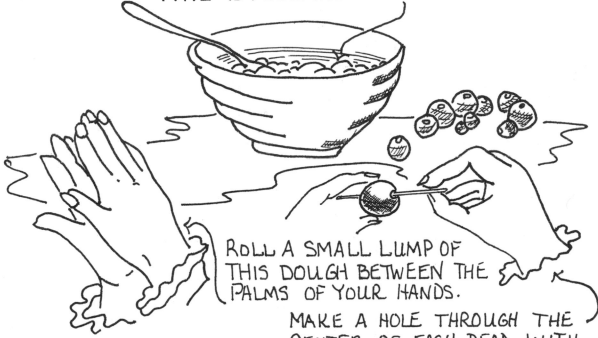

ROLL A SMALL LUMP OF THIS DOUGH BETWEEN THE PALMS OF YOUR HANDS.

MAKE A HOLE THROUGH THE CENTER OF EACH BEAD WITH A ROUND TOOTHPICK.

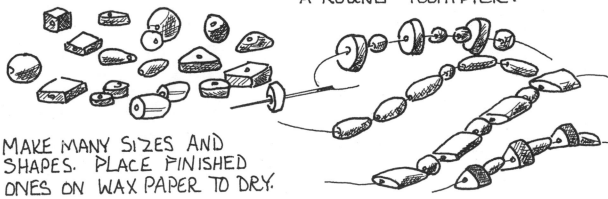

MAKE MANY SIZES AND SHAPES. PLACE FINISHED ONES ON WAX PAPER TO DRY.

STRINGING BEADS

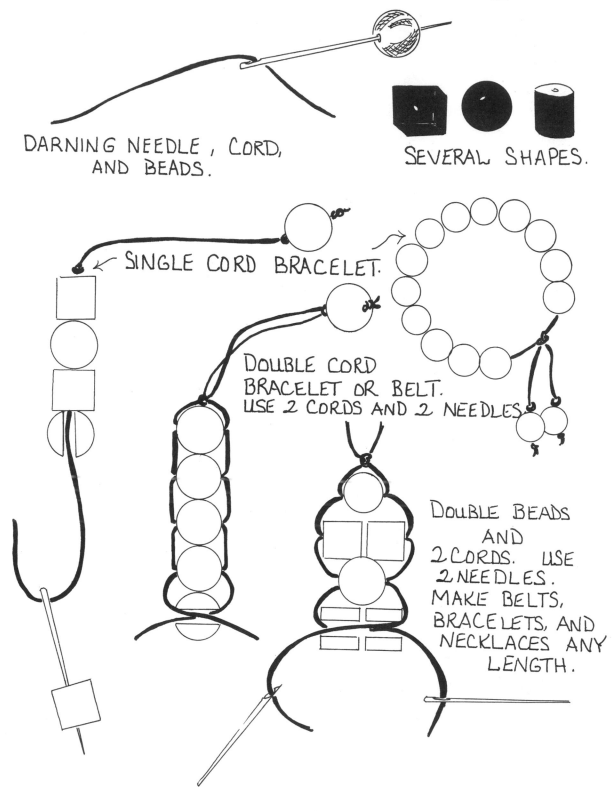

DARNING NEEDLE, CORD,
AND BEADS.

SEVERAL SHAPES.

SINGLE CORD BRACELET.

DOUBLE CORD
BRACELET OR BELT.
USE 2 CORDS AND 2 NEEDLES

DOUBLE BEADS
AND
2 CORDS. USE
2 NEEDLES.
MAKE BELTS,
BRACELETS, AND
NECKLACES ANY
LENGTH.

SEED BEADS

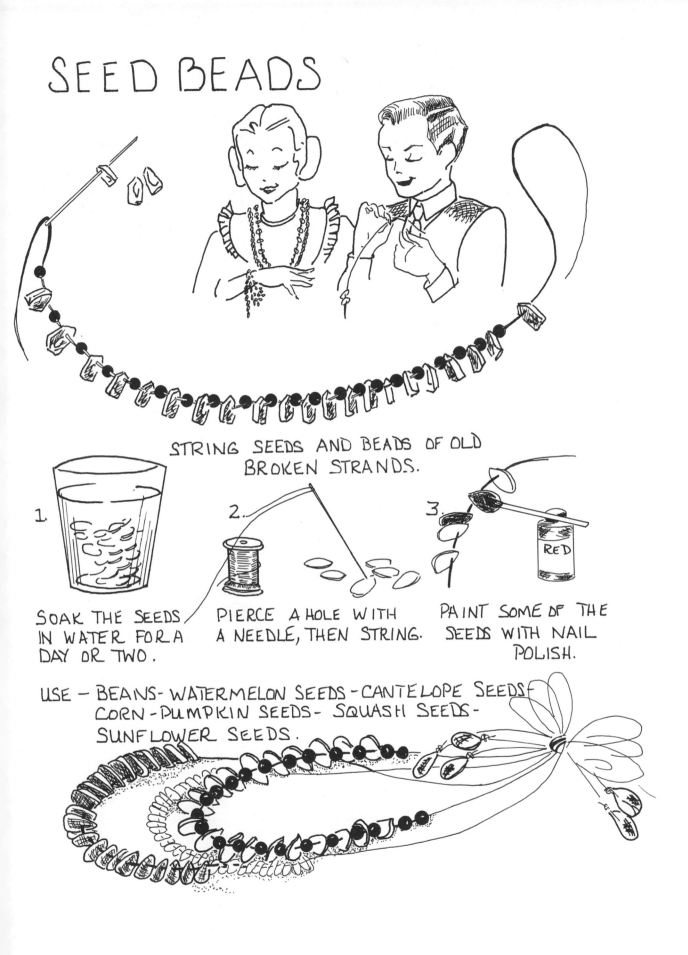

STRING SEEDS AND BEADS OF OLD BROKEN STRANDS.

1. SOAK THE SEEDS IN WATER FOR A DAY OR TWO.

2. PIERCE A HOLE WITH A NEEDLE, THEN STRING.

3. PAINT SOME OF THE SEEDS WITH NAIL POLISH.

RED

USE - BEANS - WATERMELON SEEDS - CANTELOPE SEEDS - CORN - PUMPKIN SEEDS - SQUASH SEEDS - SUNFLOWER SEEDS.

MOSAIC

Level of difficulty: *—*****

MATERIALS: Wallpaper (samples are fine), dozens of buttons, craft glue, brush; any other interesting objects such as loose beads, pearls, seeds, plastic produce baskets (all optional).

APPLICATIONS: These intricate mosaics are pleasant to view when hung on the wall opposite a bed, or place small ones on little easels on dressers or night stands.

PREPARATION BEFORE CRAFT SESSION: None

CRAFT SESSION: Let each person choose a piece of wallpaper that especially appeals to him. Brush the paper with glue, a section at a time. Then appliqué the paper with buttons. Add other objects if desired. Plastic produce baskets can be cut into rectangles. They will look like stained glass windows when glued over wallpaper that has a small design on it.

MOSAIC

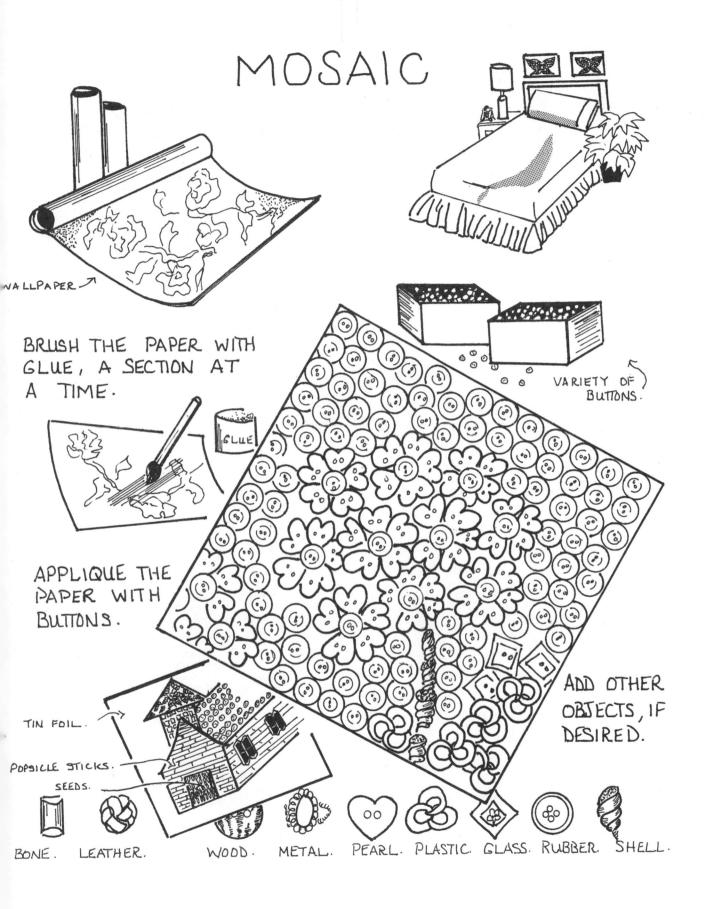

WALLPAPER

BRUSH THE PAPER WITH
GLUE, A SECTION AT
A TIME.

GLUE

VARIETY OF
BUTTONS.

APPLIQUE THE
PAPER WITH
BUTTONS.

ADD OTHER
OBJECTS, IF
DESIRED.

TIN FOIL.

POPSICLE STICKS.

SEEDS.

BONE.   LEATHER.   WOOD.   METAL.   PEARL.   PLASTIC.   GLASS.   RUBBER.   SHELL.

CACTUS TERRARIUMS

Level of difficulty: *—*****

MATERIALS: Wire clothes hangers, wire cutter, empty glass jars, plastic spoons, potting soil, sand in a variety of colors, one cactus for each terrarium, wet towels.

APPLICATIONS: A terrarium is a small garden in a glass. These colorful terrariums can decorate a windowsill or night stand and do not require regular watering by forgetful minds.

PREPARATION BEFORE CRAFT SESSION: Cut the hangers into 10-inch lengths. Divide the sands and soil into several containers so that each person has a nice selection with which to work.

CRAFT SESSION: Let each person fill a jar with layers of colored sand until it is about two-thirds full. Then using a wire hanger stick, glide the wire down the inside of the jar until it touches the bottom and lift it back along its original path. Repeat this procedure all the way around the jar to create an interesting design in the sand. Be careful not to shake the jars, or the colored sands will mix. When the design is complete, add a layer of potting soil and plant a cactus. Clean messy hands with wet towels.

CACTUS TERRARIUMS

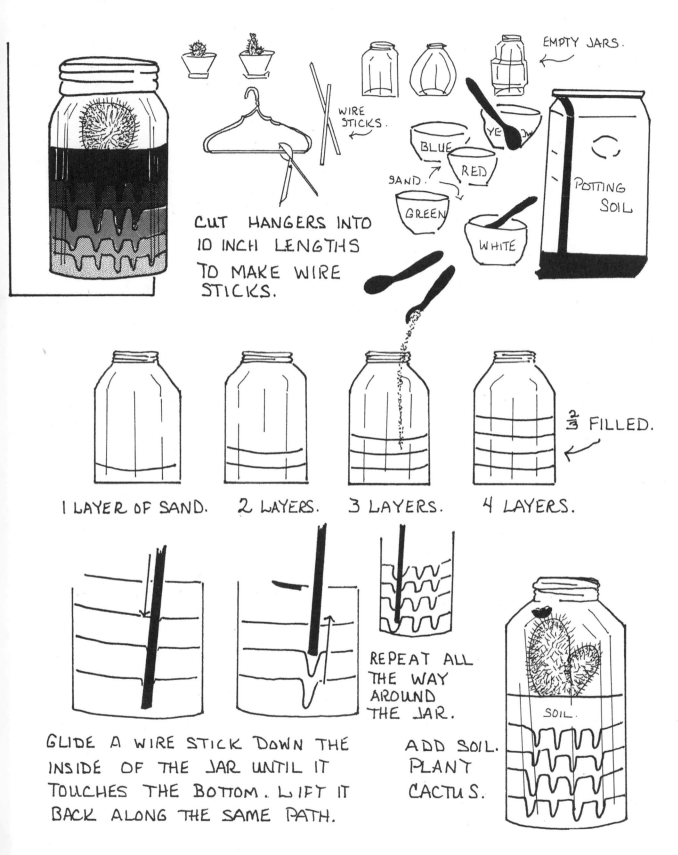

EMPTY JARS.

WIRE STICKS.

BLUE

YELLOW

RED

SAND.

GREEN

WHITE

POTTING SOIL

CUT HANGERS INTO 10 INCH LENGTHS TO MAKE WIRE STICKS.

1 LAYER OF SAND.   2 LAYERS.   3 LAYERS.   4 LAYERS.

$\frac{2}{3}$ FILLED.

GLIDE A WIRE STICK DOWN THE INSIDE OF THE JAR UNTIL IT TOUCHES THE BOTTOM. LIFT IT BACK ALONG THE SAME PATH.

REPEAT ALL THE WAY AROUND THE JAR.

ADD SOIL. PLANT CACTUS.

SOIL.

WOODEN HORSE

Level of difficulty: **—*****

MATERIALS: Fabric scraps, craft glue, scissors, spring clothespins, green yarn, wood stain, varnish, brushes, sandpaper, wood scraps, hammer, nails, jigsaw.

APPLICATIONS: Although the preparation before the craft session is somewhat tedious, the craft session itself is a lot of fun. The finished horses make an appealing toy for children or an eye-catching note or photo holder for adults. The Nursecare Nursing Center (of Charlotte, North Carolina) combined a western music day with the craft session. Each patient kept his horse as a souvenir of a happy occasion. Before the horses were attached to their bases, some of the men sanded the wood. Often men are thrilled to do this type of work even when they do not care to participate in an actual craft session.

PREPARATION BEFORE CRAFT SESSION: Using a jigsaw, cut out horses and bases. Sand the wood. Then stain and varnish the bases, horses, and clothespins (one for each horse). Attach the horses to the bases with nails and glue.

CRAFT SESSION: Using fabric scraps, cut out a mane, tail, saddle, feet and covering for the base. Using green yarn, cut out lots of grass. Glue the cloth to the horse. It is easiest to apply glue with a brush onto the horse and then lay the fabric on top of the glue. Sprinkle grass around the feet and attach the clothespin head.

WOODEN HORSE

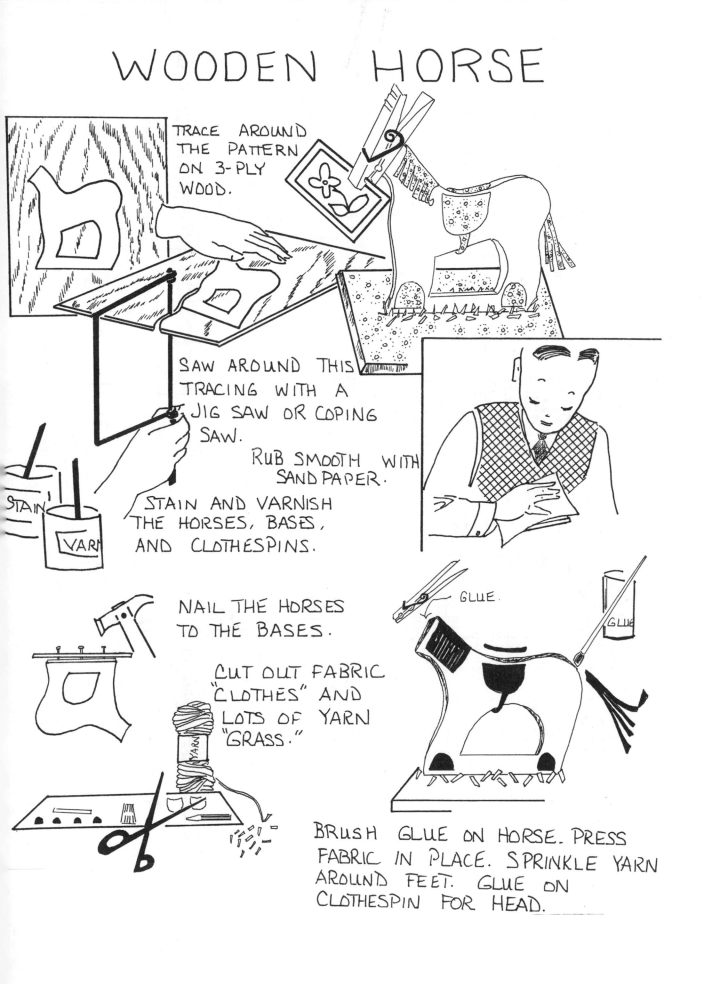

TRACE AROUND THE PATTERN ON 3-PLY WOOD.

SAW AROUND THIS TRACING WITH A JIG SAW OR COPING SAW.

RUB SMOOTH WITH SAND PAPER.

STAIN AND VARNISH THE HORSES, BASES, AND CLOTHESPINS.

NAIL THE HORSES TO THE BASES.

CUT OUT FABRIC "CLOTHES" AND LOTS OF YARN "GRASS."

GLUE.

BRUSH GLUE ON HORSE. PRESS FABRIC IN PLACE. SPRINKLE YARN AROUND FEET. GLUE ON CLOTHESPIN FOR HEAD.

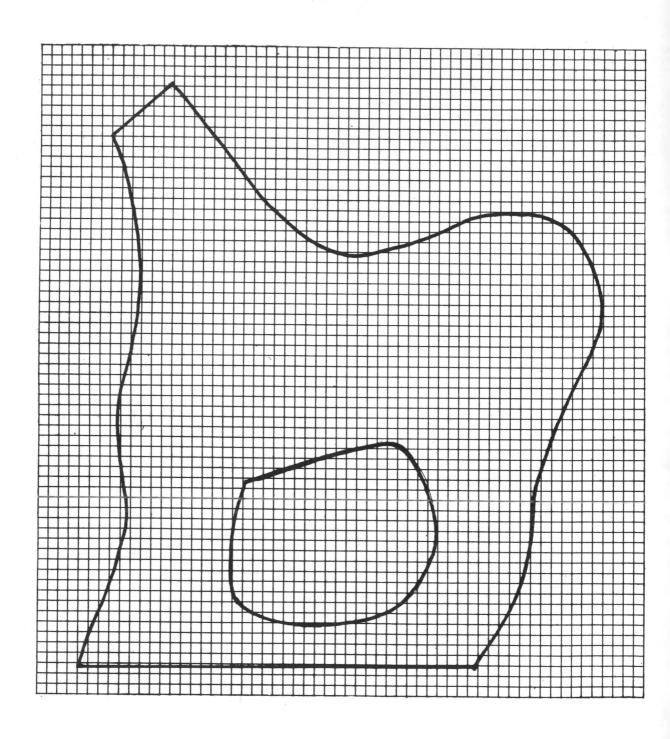

PATTERN FOR WOODEN HORSE

PATTERNS FOR WOODEN HORSE

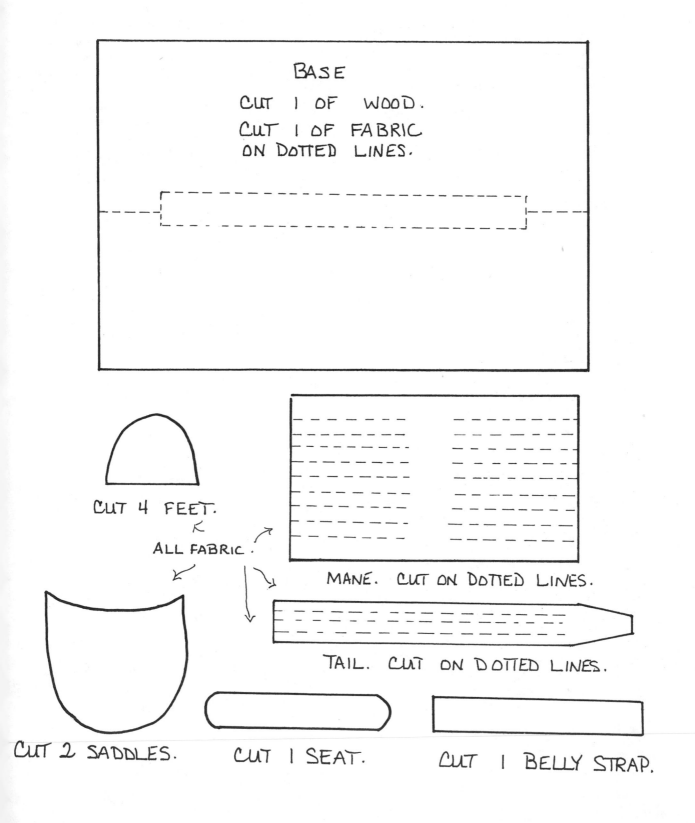

BASE

CUT 1 OF WOOD.

CUT 1 OF FABRIC
ON DOTTED LINES.

CUT 4 FEET.

ALL FABRIC.

MANE. CUT ON DOTTED LINES.

TAIL. CUT ON DOTTED LINES.

CUT 2 SADDLES.

CUT 1 SEAT.

CUT 1 BELLY STRAP.

MATCHING FABRIC NOTECARDS

Level of difficulty: *—*****

MATERIALS: Two yards, unbleached muslin, felt marking pens in a variety of colors, pinking shears, glue, drawing paper, envelopes, scissors, ball point pen, rubber bands, or string.

APPLICATIONS: These cards become *matched* when the very large piece of decorated cloth is cut into many small pieces. These notecards are always handy for patients to give to special visitors or to write friends on special occasions.

PREPARATION BEFORE CRAFT SESSION: Cut dozens of pieces of drawing paper which, when folded in half, will fit the envelopes you have for the notes. On the bottom of the back of each folded note, print "made by ————." (I used the name of our nursing home, but you may prefer to insert individual names.) I also use beige drawing paper to match the muslin, but this is not necessary.

CRAFT SESSION: Using felt pens in a variety of colors, have each person decorate the cloth until it is solidly covered with color. Hit the cloth at random to make dozens of dots or dashes; scribble in large or small circles; draw pictures; sign names; use imagination. The idea is for everyone to contribute to the overall coloring of the fabric. Then cut the material with pinking shears to fit each folded note. Glue the fabric to the note. Stack the notes with an equal set of envelopes. Secure the notes and envelopes with rubber bands or string.

MATCHING FABRIC NOTECARDS

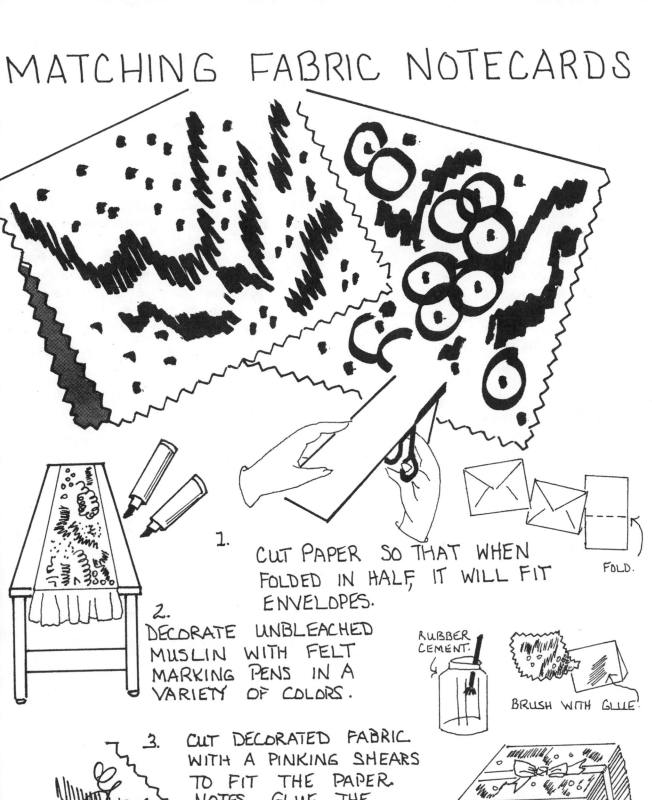

1. CUT PAPER SO THAT WHEN FOLDED IN HALF, IT WILL FIT ENVELOPES.

FOLD.

2. DECORATE UNBLEACHED MUSLIN WITH FELT MARKING PENS IN A VARIETY OF COLORS.

RUBBER CEMENT.

BRUSH WITH GLUE.

3. CUT DECORATED FABRIC WITH A PINKING SHEARS TO FIT THE PAPER NOTES. GLUE THE FABRIC TO THE PAPER.

4. AND TIE STACKS OF NOTECARDS AND ENVELOPES.

DRESSER SCARVES

Level of difficulty: *—*****

MATERIALS: Unbleached muslin (or any inexpensive, pastel, unpatterned fabric), scissors, wax crayons, iron, wax paper, masking tape.

APPLICATIONS: The illustration shows you how to make a dresser scarf by applying this method of decoration. After you have learned the method, you can make other decorated textiles such as placemats, dollhouse curtains, or handkerchiefs.

PREPARATION BEFORE CRAFT SESSION: Pull the threads, one at a time, along each edge to make the fringe; or hem the scarves with a blanket stitch. Draw a pattern on the scarves with a pencil. Then, using the masking tape, tape each doily to the table in front of each person so that it will not slide around.

CRAFT SESSION: Have each person color the entire design with wax crayons, using any colors they wish. Better results are obtained if they color with the weave of the material, namely, across and lengthwise. Be sure to put each person's name on his scarf before untaping it. Then set the crayon yourself by melting it into the cloth so that it does not wash out or wear off. To do this, place a piece of wax paper over the crayoned doily and press it with a very warm iron. *Be careful* that the people with whom you are working cannot reach the iron or its cord.

DRESSER SCARVES

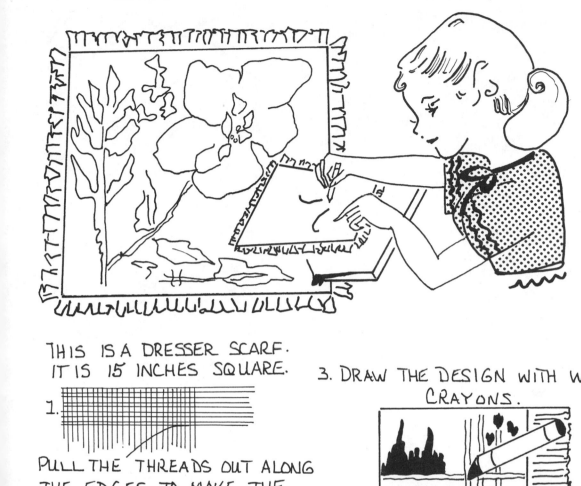

THIS IS A DRESSER SCARF.
IT IS 15 INCHES SQUARE.

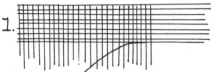

PULL THE THREADS OUT ALONG
THE EDGES TO MAKE THE
FRINGE.

2. TAPE THE SCARF TO THE
TABLE SO IT WON'T SLIDE.

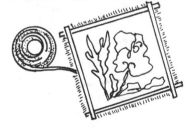

3. DRAW THE DESIGN WITH WAX
CRAYONS.

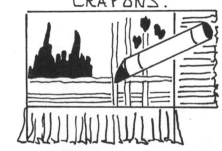

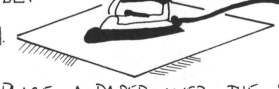

4.

PLACE A PAPER OVER THE SCARF
AND PRESS WITH A VERY WARM IRON.

5. THESE ARE OTHER
IDEAS.

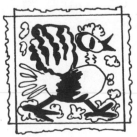

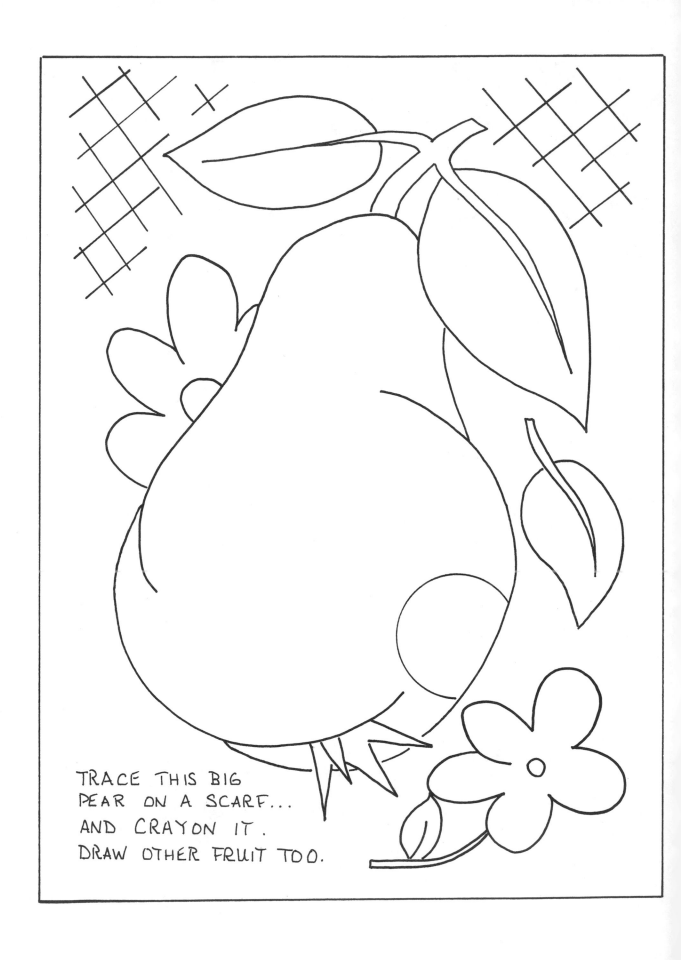

TRACE THIS BIG
PEAR ON A SCARF...
AND CRAYON IT.
DRAW OTHER FRUIT TOO.

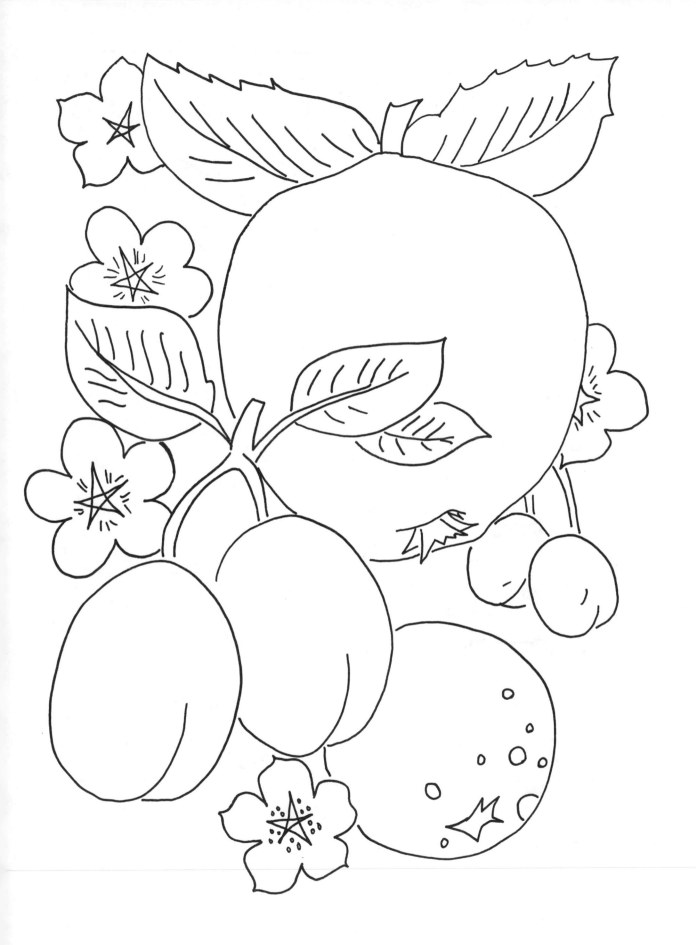

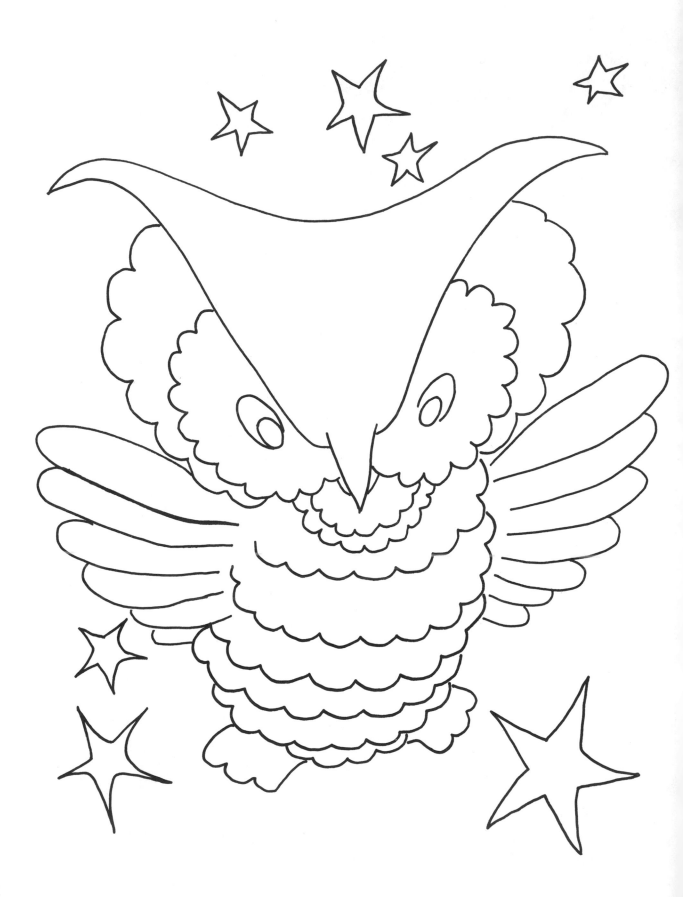

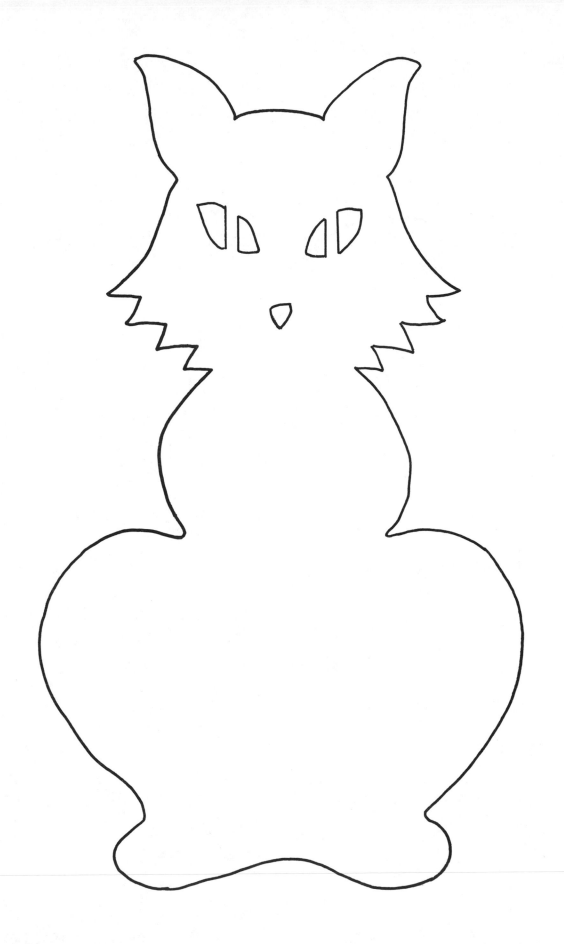

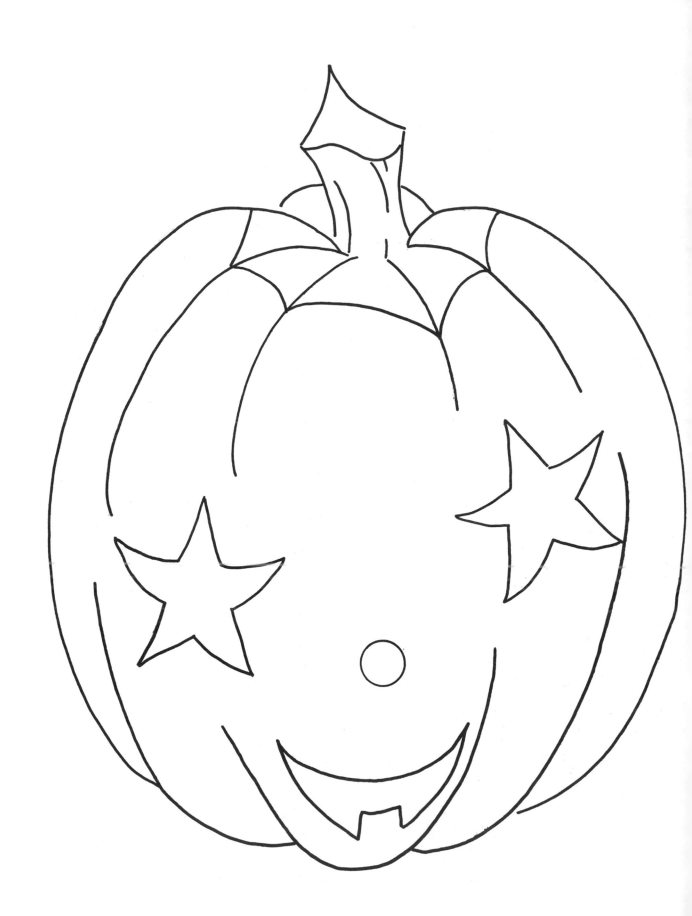

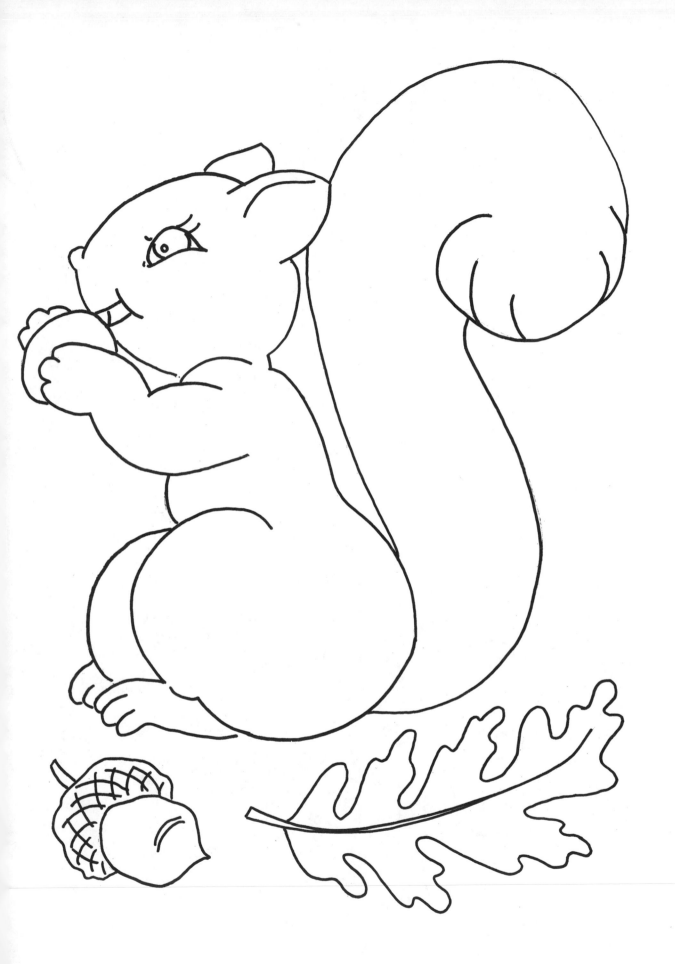

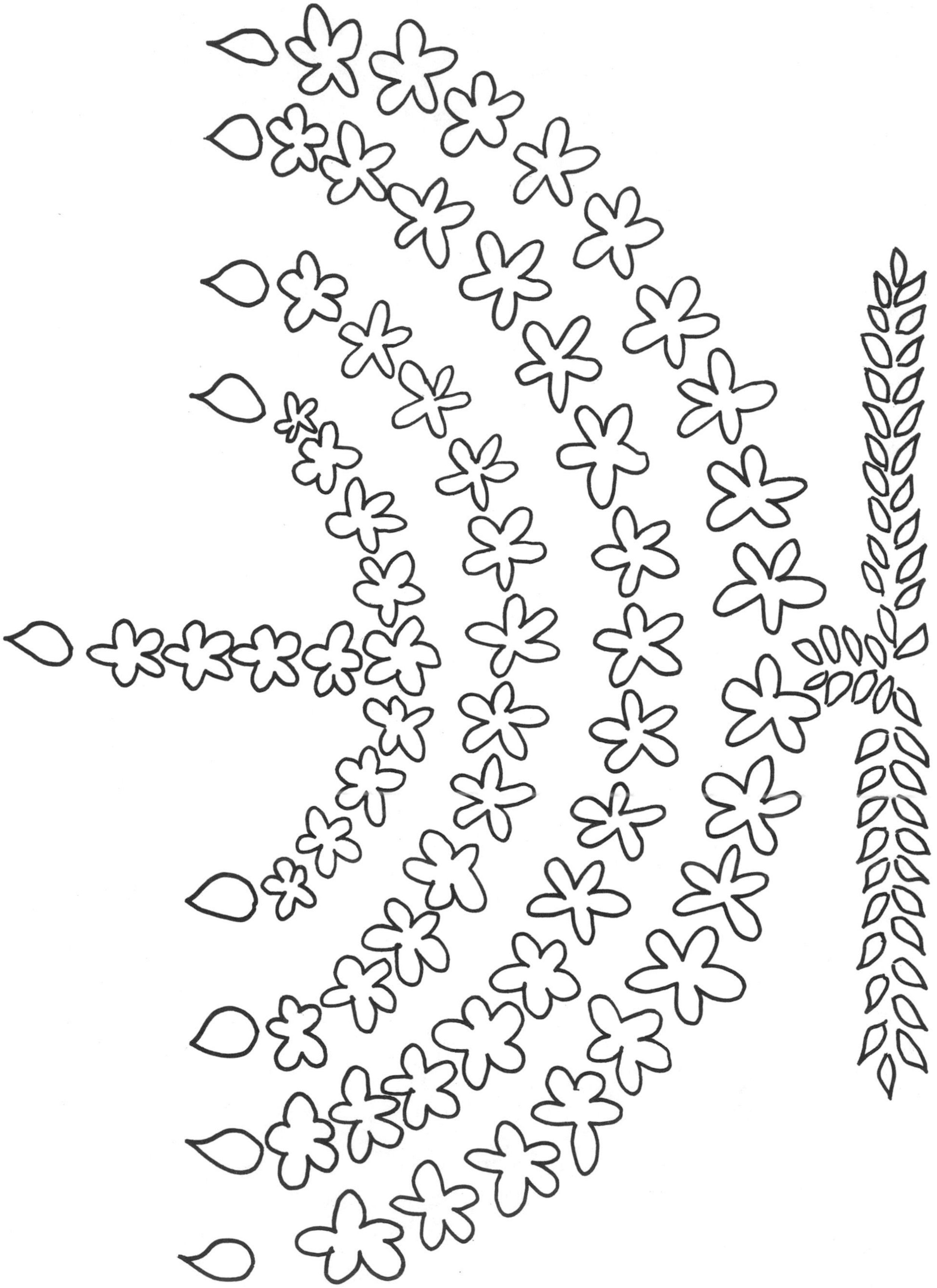

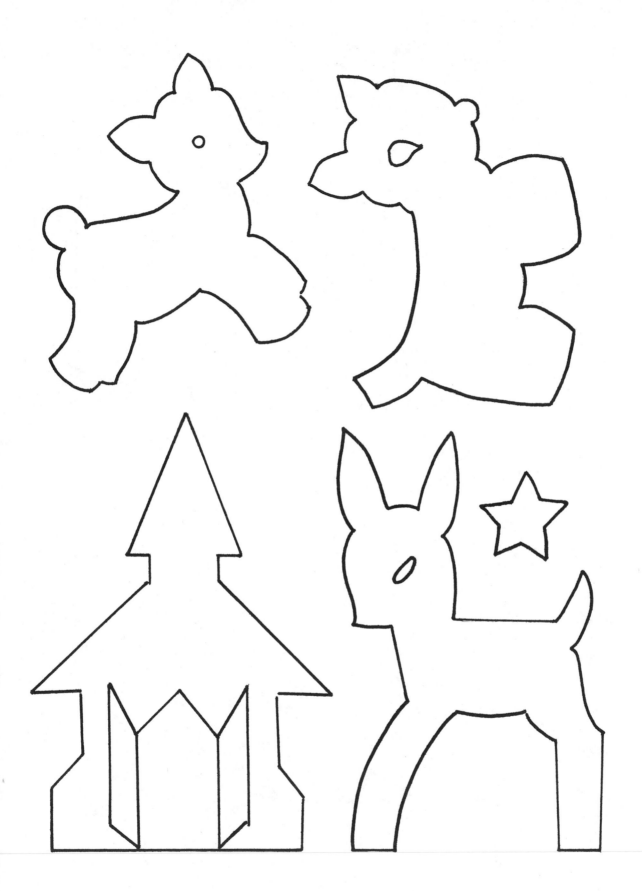

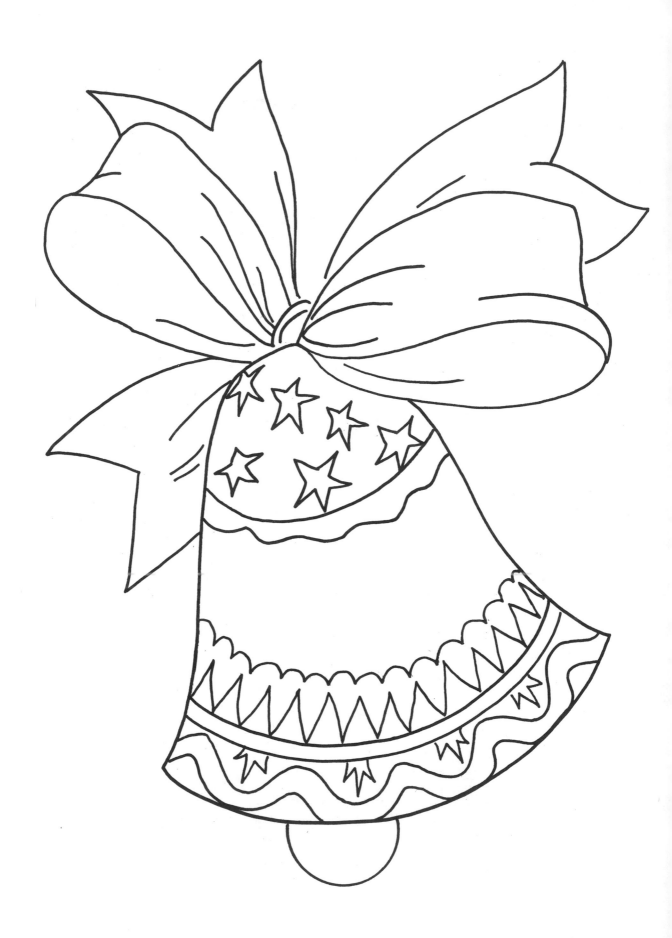

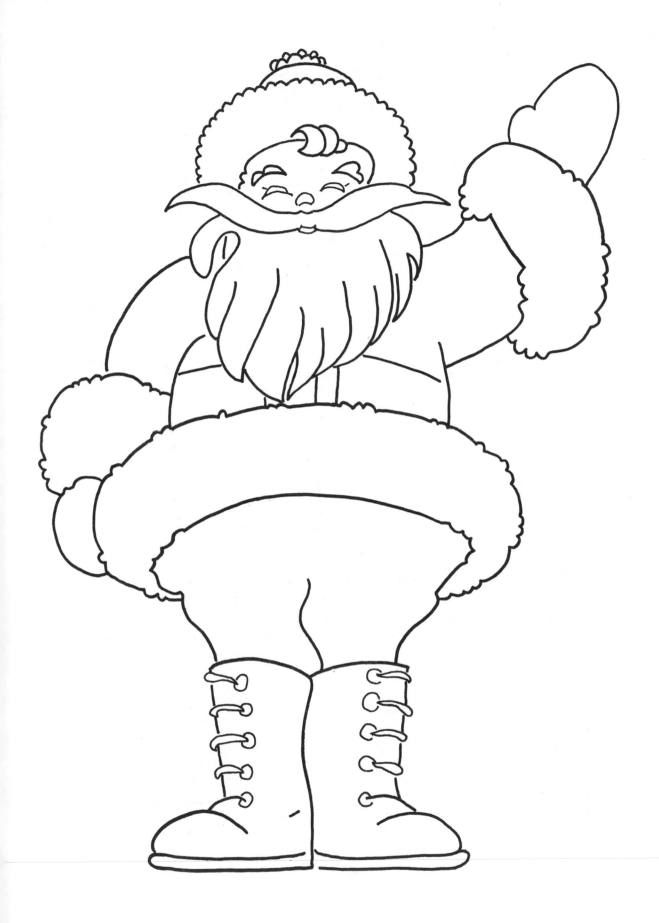

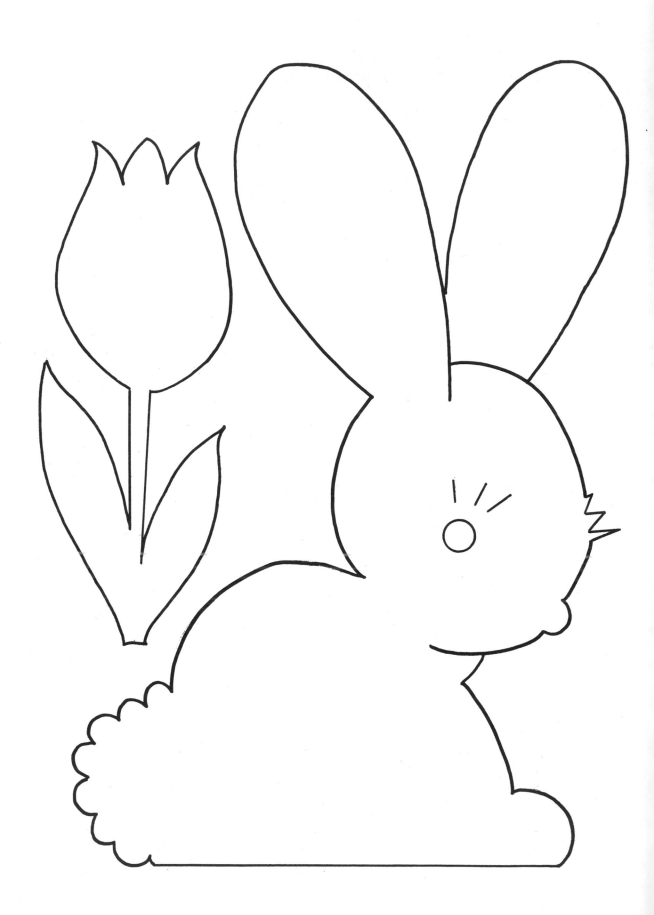

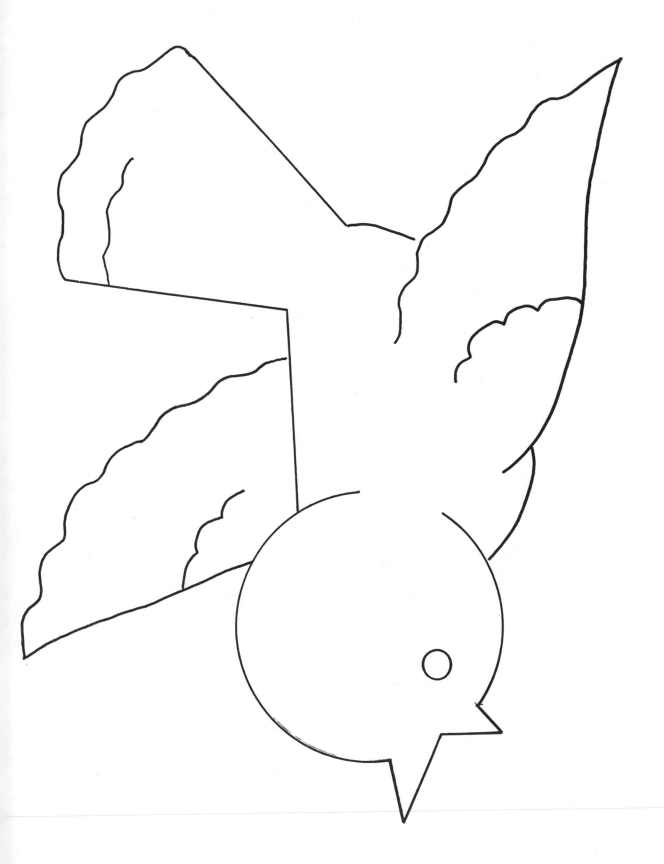

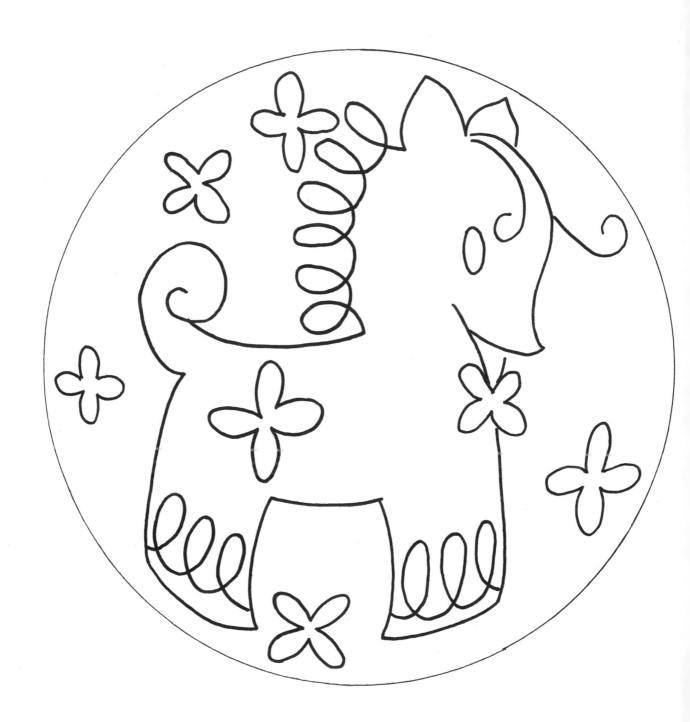

WALL POCKET

Level of difficulty: *—***

MATERIALS: Glue stick, scissors, paper plates, felt marking pens in a variety of colors, paper punch, paper fasteners, pencil, yarn, tacks.

APPLICATIONS: These wall pockets are nice to save special letters or pretty clippings from magazines to use for other projects.

PREPARATION BEFORE CRAFT SESSION: Cut enough plates in half to make one half for each whole plate. Each person should have one whole plate and one half plate. Draw simple designs with a pencil on the back of the half plates. Using glue stick, secure a whole plate (right side up) and half plate (wrong side up) in front of each person.

CRAFT SESSION: Have each person decorate and color the plates using the felt pens. You may substitute tempera paints or crayon. Remove the plates from the table. Hold the half plate onto the whole plate and punch five holes along the edge. Fasten the plates together with paper fasteners through the holes you have punched. Punch two more holes at the top, each about 1½ inches from the center. Tie a piece of yarn through these holes so that the plates can be hung up and used for a wall pocket. See that each person gets a tack and help, if necessary, to hang his pocket.

WALL POCKET

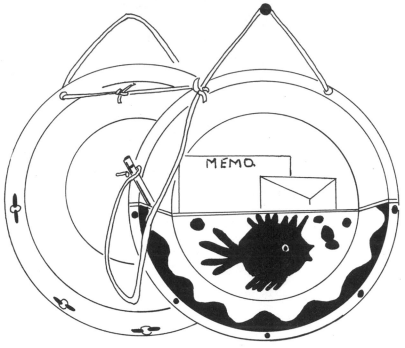
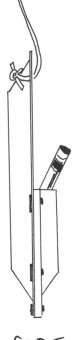

BACK.

FRONT.

SIDE.

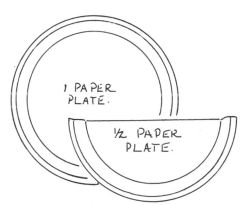

1 PAPER PLATE.

½ PAPER PLATE.

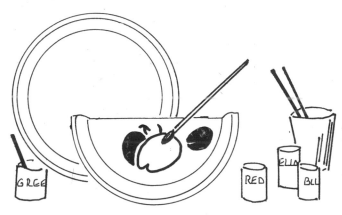

GREE

RED   ELLA   BLU

PUT STRING THROUGH HOLES.

PAINT THE BACK OF THE HALF PLATE AND THE FRONT OF THE WHOLE PLATE.

USE TEMPERA PAINT OR FELT PENS.

PUNCH HOLES AND FASTEN TOGETHER WITH PAPER FASTENERS.

FASTENER OPEN ON BACK.

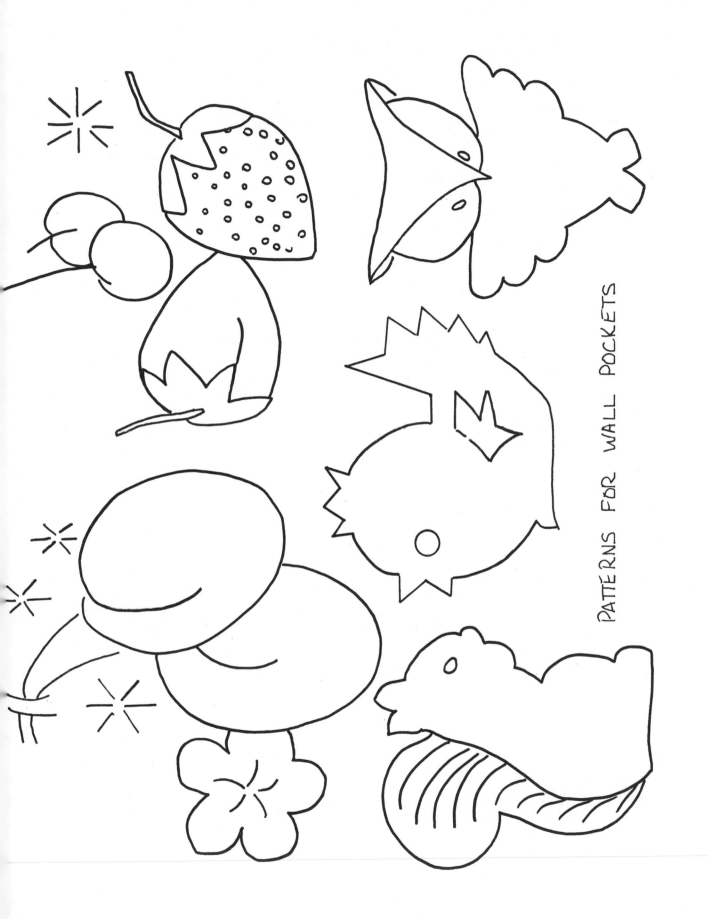

PATTERNS FOR WALL POCKETS

PATCHWORK POTS

Level of difficulty: *—*****

MATERIALS: Clay or plastic flower pots in a variety of sizes, craft glue, brushes, water, empty plastic containers, pinking shears, fabric scraps, ric rac (very narrow, preferably), pen, varnish or craft glaze (optional).

APPLICATIONS: These patchwork pots are absolutely beautiful and foolproof. Gingham or calico squares do not have to be matched to be attractive. However, many older persons enjoy working out intricate designs with the fabric reminiscent of quilting parties in earlier years. Cuttings of rapid growing plants (baby tears and grape ivy) can be planted in the finished pots. Relatives and friends admire the work and often place special orders for pots in particular colors. Favorite combinations were red, yellow, and green or red, white, and blue.

Even a partially blind person can paint glue on a pot, and a partner can arrange the fabric squares on the pot. Shaking hands find this to be a confidence building project.

PREPARATION BEFORE CRAFT SESSION: Mix craft glue with a little water until it is the consistency of white glue. Using a pinking shears, cut out dozens of fabric squares approximately 1 inch by 1 inch.

CRAFT SESSION: Put each person's name on the bottom of his pot. This will come in handy when you return the pot with a plant in it. Brush glue on the pot, a section at a time. Arrange the squares attractively on the glue. Be certain to overlap each square slightly so that the pot will not show through the cloth. Then trim the pot with ric rac both vertically around the pot and also around the circumference of the upper and lower rim and bottom of the pot.

After the pot dries, apply several coats of the glue and water mixture over the entire pot, letting it dry between each application. If you like, seal the pot with varnish or shellac or a commercially available craft glaze. *Be sure* to do this *away* from patients, as the fumes may be harmful.

PATCHWORK POTS

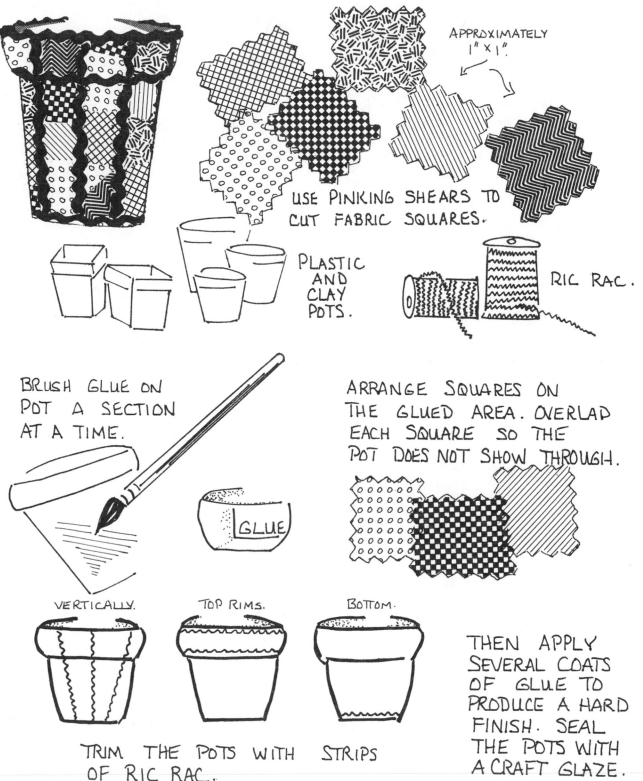

USE PINKING SHEARS TO CUT FABRIC SQUARES.

APPROXIMATELY 1" X 1"

PLASTIC AND CLAY POTS.

RIC RAC.

BRUSH GLUE ON POT A SECTION AT A TIME.

GLUE

ARRANGE SQUARES ON THE GLUED AREA. OVERLAP EACH SQUARE SO THE POT DOES NOT SHOW THROUGH.

VERTICALLY.

TOP RIMS.

BOTTOM.

TRIM THE POTS WITH OF RIC RAC.

STRIPS

THEN APPLY SEVERAL COATS OF GLUE TO PRODUCE A HARD FINISH. SEAL THE POTS WITH A CRAFT GLAZE.

WASTE BASKETS

Level of difficulty: *—*****

MATERIALS: Five-gallon ice cream cartons, fabric, craft glue, brushes, water, empty plastic containers, ric rac or other trim, pinking shears, plastic bags, varnish or craft glaze (optional).

APPLICATIONS: These waste baskets are an attractive addition to any room. Men seem to like this project because it is not dainty. Choose masculine prints.

PREPARATION BEFORE CRAFT SESSION: Using a pinking shears, cut strips of fabric 2 inches by 13 inches. Mix craft glue with water until it is the consistency of white glue.

CRAFT SESSION: Brush the glue on the empty container a section at a time. Arrange the strips of fabric attractively on the glue. You might like to place the strips diagonally across the container. Be certain to overlap each strip slightly so that the container will not show through the cloth. Then trim the basket with ric rac around the top and bottom edges. After the basket dries, apply several coats of the glue and water mixture over the entire container, letting it dry between each application. If you like, seal the basket with varnish or shellac or a commercially available craft glaze. *Be sure* to do this *away* from patients, as the fumes may be harmful.

WASTE BASKETS

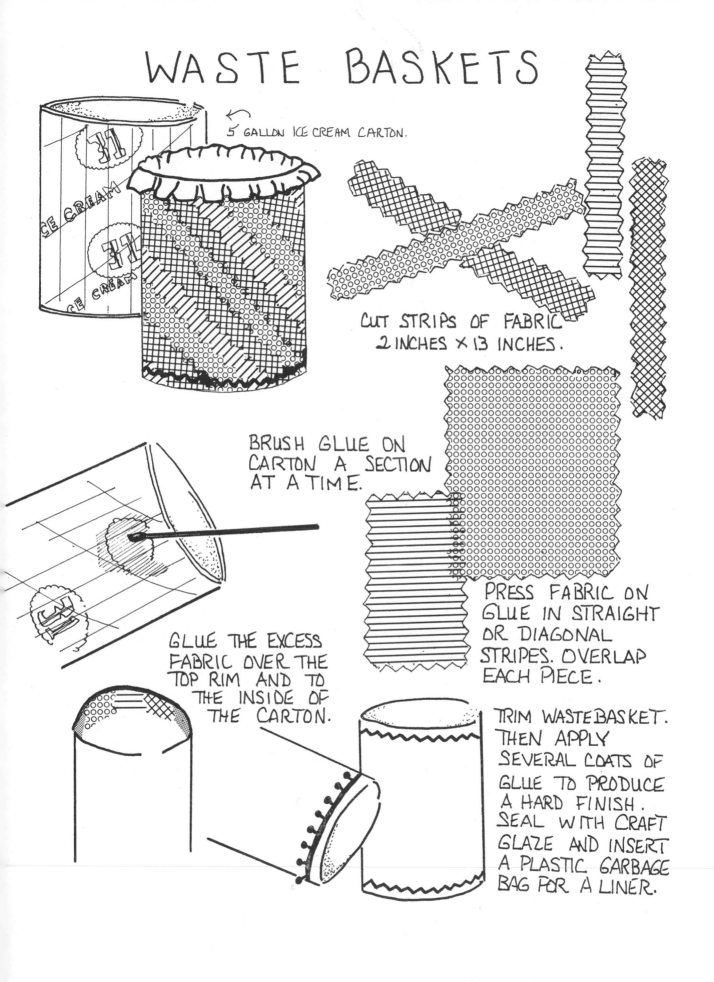

5 GALLON ICE CREAM CARTON.

CUT STRIPS OF FABRIC
2 INCHES × 13 INCHES.

BRUSH GLUE ON
CARTON A SECTION
AT A TIME.

PRESS FABRIC ON
GLUE IN STRAIGHT
OR DIAGONAL
STRIPES. OVERLAP
EACH PIECE.

GLUE THE EXCESS
FABRIC OVER THE
TOP RIM AND TO
THE INSIDE OF
THE CARTON.

TRIM WASTEBASKET.
THEN APPLY
SEVERAL COATS OF
GLUE TO PRODUCE
A HARD FINISH.
SEAL WITH CRAFT
GLAZE AND INSERT
A PLASTIC GARBAGE
BAG FOR A LINER.

CROSS-STITCH

Level of difficulty: ***—*****

MATERIALS: Checked gingham, embroidery floss in a variety of colors, needles, scissors, thimble (optional), pencil, embroidery hoop or wooden frame, tacks.

APPLICATIONS: Many people look forward to senior years as a time to do creative stitchery. And then illness strikes and limits the use of an arm. The frame shown in the illustration can be anchored to a table top or wheelchair so that a person with the use of only one arm can cross-stitch. Use cross-stitch designs for aprons, towels, pillow cases, scarves, and pictures.

PREPARATION BEFORE CRAFT SESSION: Cut gingham into appropriate sizes for articles to be made. Finish the edges with a blanket stitch. Use large gingham print for those people who have difficulty seeing small squares. Using a pencil, prepare a design on the gingham. Then place the fabric in an embroidery hoop or secure it across a wooden frame with tacks. (Some people may prefer to create their own designs.)

CRAFT SESSION: Help each person choose an article he wants to stitch and thread needles with appropriate colors. Then cross-stitch until the article is finished. Help him knot and cut the thread. Perhaps he knows how to stitch initials on the completed article.

CROSS-STITCH

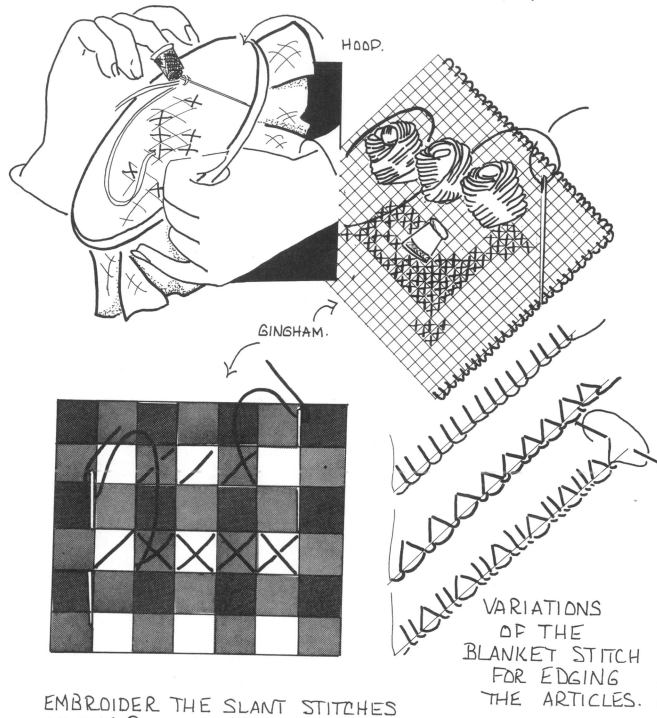

HOOP.

GINGHAM.

VARIATIONS OF THE BLANKET STITCH FOR EDGING THE ARTICLES.

EMBROIDER THE SLANT STITCHES OF ONE ROW IN ONE DIRECTION. THESE ARE CROSSED BY A SECOND ROW OF STITCHES IN THE OPPOSITE.

CROSS-STITCH FRAME

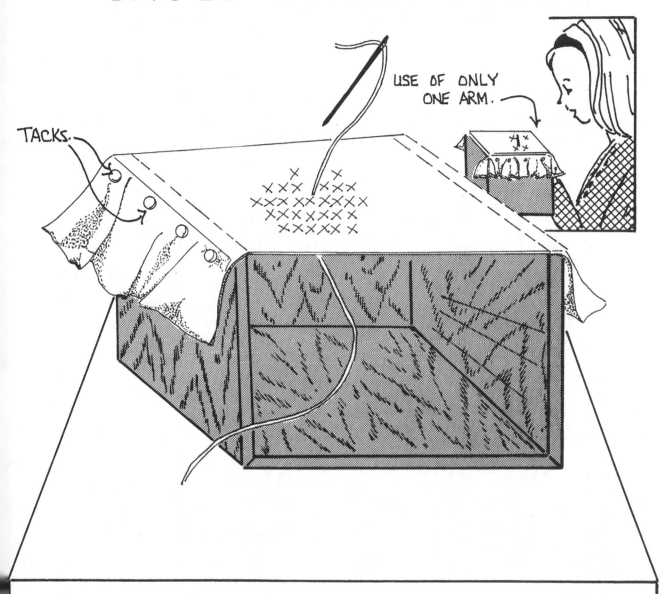

TACKS.

USE OF ONLY ONE ARM.

SEWING FRAME IS 4-SIDED WOODEN
BOX. THE TOP AND FRONT ARE
OPEN. SECURE CLOTH ACROSS TOP
OPENING TIGHTLY WITH TACKS.

CROSS-STITCH PATTERN

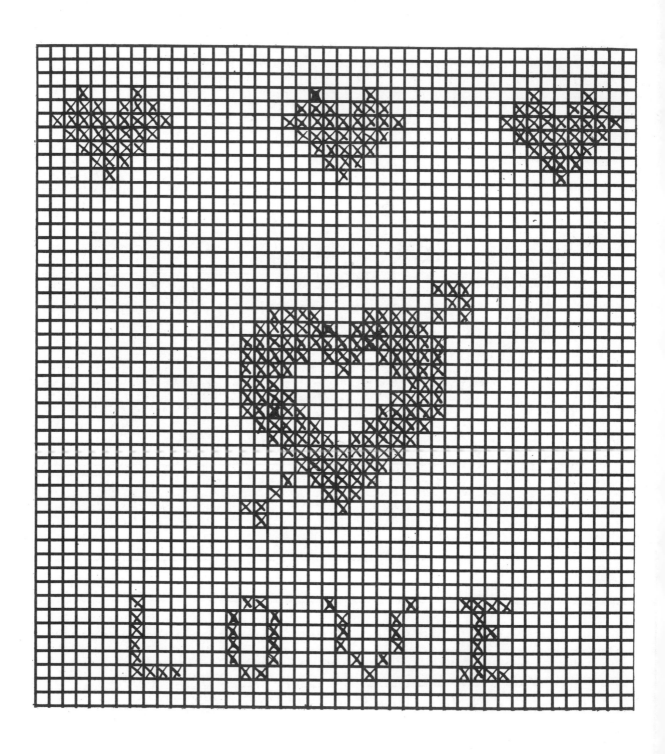

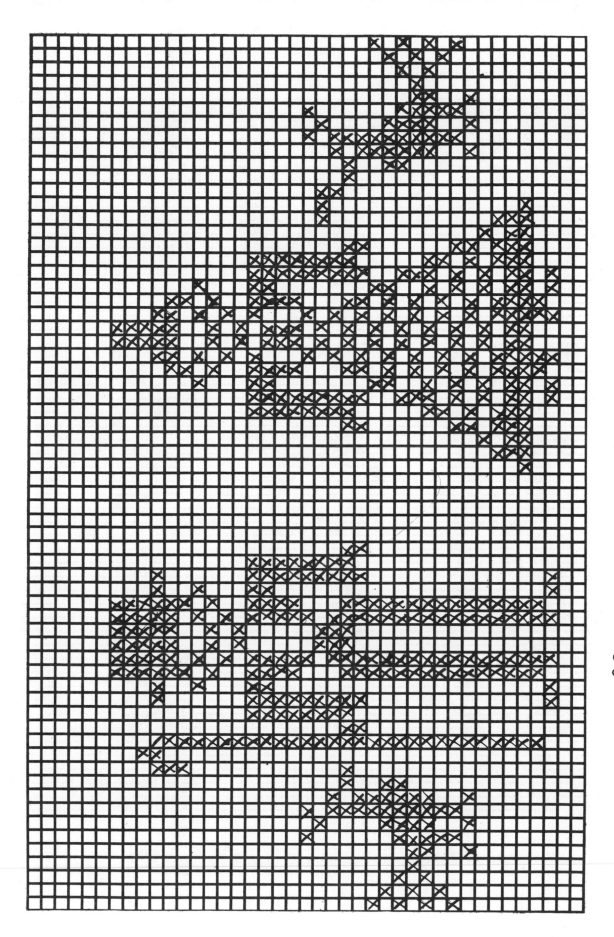

CROSS - STITCH PATTERN

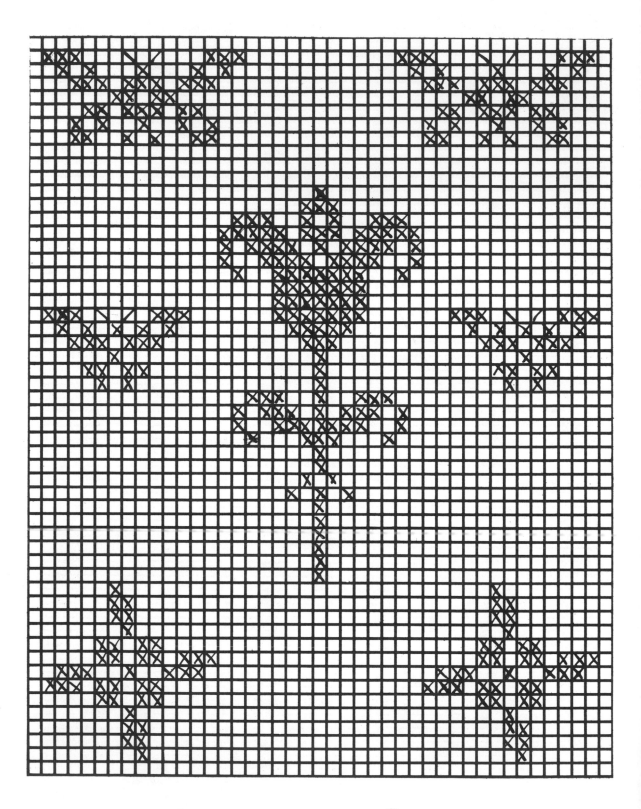

CROSS-STITCH PATTERN

CHAPTER FOUR

Craft Projects for Use by Other Patients

DECORATED WALKING STICKS

Level of difficulty: ***—*****

MATERIALS: Smooth branches or limbs about 4 feet in length, acrylic paints, brushes, newspaper or white adhesive tape, felt marking pens in a variety of colors.

APPLICATIONS: Many people enjoy using a walking stick when strolling through the garden, around corridors, or on field trips to shopping centers or special events.

PREPARATION BEFORE CRAFT SESSION: Prepare some branches for those who find paints too messy. To do this, wrap adhesive tape around sections of the branches. You will be able to see the colors of the pens on these white areas.

CRAFT SESSION: Place the branches over newspaper and make designs with paints. Try using a knot as a nose of a face. Use felt marking pens to color the adhesive tape, if you do not like to work with paint.

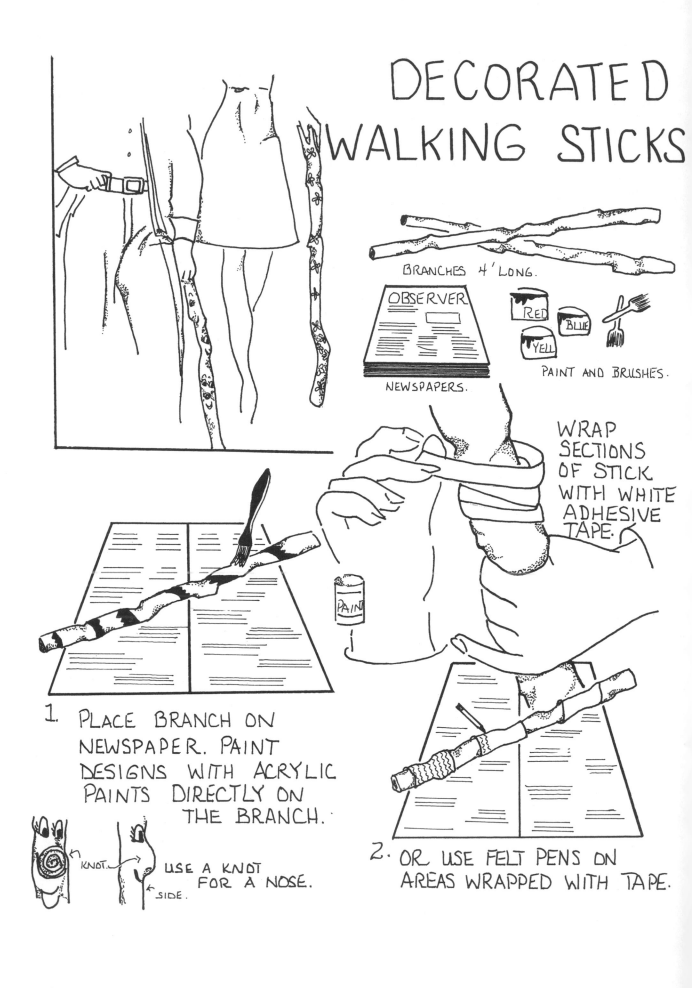

DECORATED WALKING STICKS

BRANCHES 4' LONG.

OBSERVER

NEWSPAPERS.

RED
BLUE
YELL

PAINT AND BRUSHES.

WRAP SECTIONS OF STICK WITH WHITE ADHESIVE TAPE.

PAINT

1. PLACE BRANCH ON NEWSPAPER. PAINT DESIGNS WITH ACRYLIC PAINTS DIRECTLY ON THE BRANCH.

KNOT.
USE A KNOT FOR A NOSE.
SIDE.

2. OR USE FELT PENS ON AREAS WRAPPED WITH TAPE.

IDEAS FOR DECORATED WALKING STICK

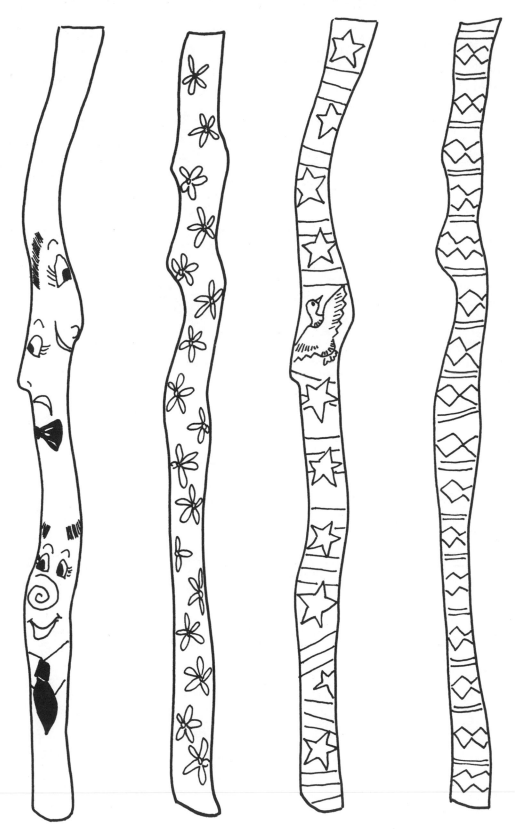

PILLOWS

Level of difficulty: *—*****

MATERIALS: Fabric scraps, scissors, needle, thread, stuffing, several large sheets of paper, pencil, iron, ironing board, pins.

APPLICATIONS: Throw pillows are good for back support in wheelchairs or neck support in beds. Try making thin pillows for cushions to sit upon. It is nice to have those who can sew well make the pillow covers and let senile or blind patients then stuff the pillows. Choose fabrics you think friends would enjoy.

PREPARATION BEFORE CRAFT SESSION: Make paper patterns for the pillows. You can make rectangles, squares, circles, or animal shapes. Pin the pattern to the fabric, and cut out two pieces of cloth the same shape and size. Press the fabric pieces with a warm iron. *Be sure* to keep the cord and iron *away* from patients.

CRAFT SESSION: Place the front of the pillow, design face up, on a table and lay the pillow back on top, making certain that all the sides and corners match as exactly as possible. Be sure that the wrong side of each piece of fabric is on the outside, as you will be turning the pillow inside out. Pin the two pieces of cloth securely together. Using a needle and thread, stitch around the pillow about ⅝ inch from the edge, leaving a 6-inch opening for the stuffing. Clip any corners close to the stitching as shown in the illustration. Remove the pins. Then turn the pillow inside out. Poke the corners out until the shape is accurate again. Stuff the pillow, being sure to push the stuffing (polyester, cotton, old nylons, or fabric bits) into the corners. Fill the pillow as full as you like; then pin the opening closed and sew it by hand. Shake the pillow to distribute the stuffing evenly.

PILLOWS

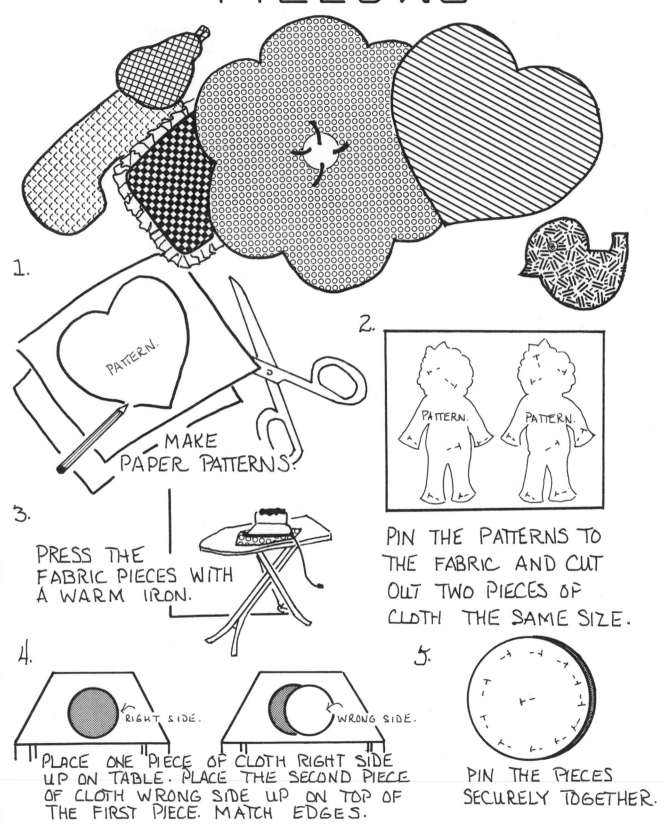

1. MAKE PAPER PATTERNS.

PATTERN.

2. PIN THE PATTERNS TO THE FABRIC AND CUT OUT TWO PIECES OF CLOTH THE SAME SIZE.

PATTERN. PATTERN.

3. PRESS THE FABRIC PIECES WITH A WARM IRON.

4. PLACE ONE PIECE OF CLOTH RIGHT SIDE UP ON TABLE. PLACE THE SECOND PIECE OF CLOTH WRONG SIDE UP ON TOP OF THE FIRST PIECE. MATCH EDGES.

RIGHT SIDE.

WRONG SIDE.

5. PIN THE PIECES SECURELY TOGETHER.

PILLOWS

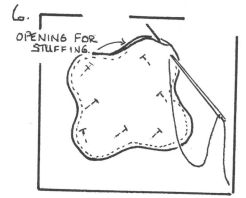

OPENING FOR STUFFING.

STITCH AROUND THE PILLOW ABOUT 5/8 INCH FROM THE EDGE, LEAVING A 6 INCH OPENING.

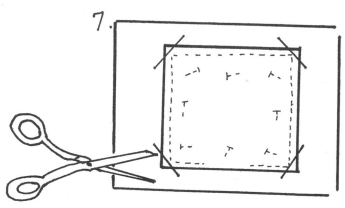

CLIP CORNERS CLOSE TO THE STITCHING. REMOVE THE PINS.

8.

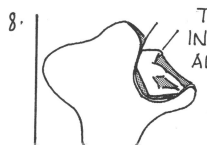

TURN THE PILLOW INSIDE OUT. POKE ALL THE CORNERS TO SHAPE THE PILLOW.

9.

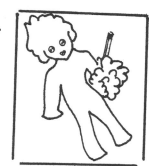

STUFF THE PILLOW. BE SURE TO GET INTO ALL THE CORNERS.

10.

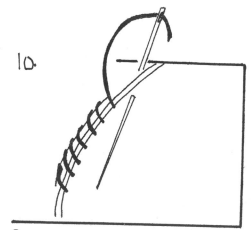

PIN THE OPENING AND SEW IT CLOSED.

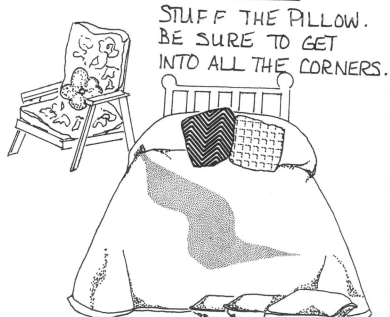

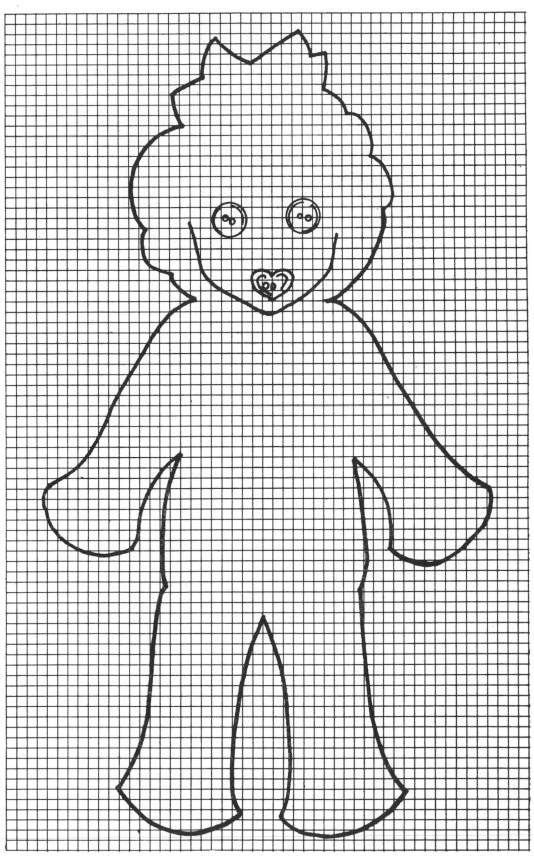

ENLARGE THIS PILLOW PATTERN.

HANGING BASKET

Level of difficulty: ****—*****

MATERIALS: Raffia or twine, buttons or beads, metal rings, scissors, cup hook or bracket.

APPLICATIONS: This hanging basket is like a large net and will hold different shapes and sizes of containers for plants and flowers. A basket makes an especially nice gift for a friend who does not have enough table space to display his plants.

PREPARATION BEFORE CRAFT SESSION: Cut raffia or twine into 48-inch lengths. Fasten eight or twelve lengths of raffia to a metal or bone ring as shown in the illustration.

CRAFT SESSION: Start weaving at the bottom of the basket. To do this, take one end of the raffia loop and one end of the loop next to it. String these through a button or bead until they are about 2 inches from the ring. Continue this process around the ring. Now you have one row of buttons or beads around the ring. String the next row of buttons with the opposite raffia lengths 3 inches from the first row of buttons. Repeat another row 3 inches farther on the raffia; and, if you wish the basket still larger, add another row. Tie all the ends to hold them together at the top. Hook this hanger over a cup hook or bracket.

HANGING BASKET

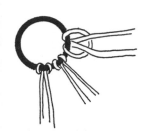

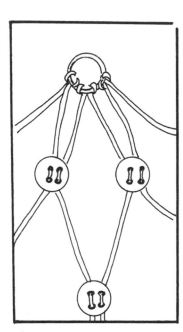

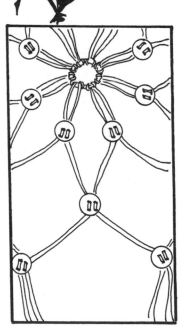

FASTEN 8 OR 12 LENGTHS OF RAFFIA TO A METAL RING. RAFFIA FOLDED SHOULD BE 24".

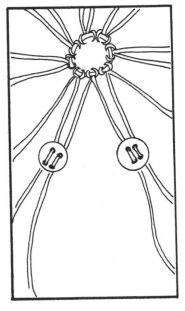

TAKE ONE END OF ONE RAFFIA LOOP AND ONE END OF THE LOOP NEXT TO IT. STRING THESE THROUGH A BUTTON 2" FROM THE RING. CONTINUE AROUND THE RING.

THEN STRING THE NEXT ROW OF BUTTONS WITH THE OPPOSITE RAFFIA LENGTHS 3" FROM THE FIRST ROW OF BUTTONS.

REPEAT ANOTHER ROW 3" FARTHER ON THE RAFFIA.

WIND CHIMES

Level of difficulty: ***—*****

MATERIALS: Round-headed clothespins, plastic lids, ribbon, colored string, scissors, nail, cup hook.

APPLICATIONS: Musical wind chimes which sing in the breeze are a welcome addition to any patio area. Try hanging the chimes over an open window. Bed ridden patients like to watch the movement and hear the music of the wind chimes.

PREPARATION BEFORE CRAFT SESSION: Using a nail, punch ten pairs of holes in a plastic lid about 1 inch apart as shown in the illustration. Cut ten 15-inch pieces of string for each lid.

CRAFT SESSION: Push a piece of string up through one hole in the lid and down through the other. Make a knot in the end of the string too large to pull back through the hole. Pull the string tightly. Tie the other end of the string around the neck of a clothespin. Repeat this process until there are ten clothespins hanging about the same height from the lid. Then poke a hole in the center of the lid and tie a pretty ribbon through it for hanging the chimes from a cup hook.

WIND CHIMES

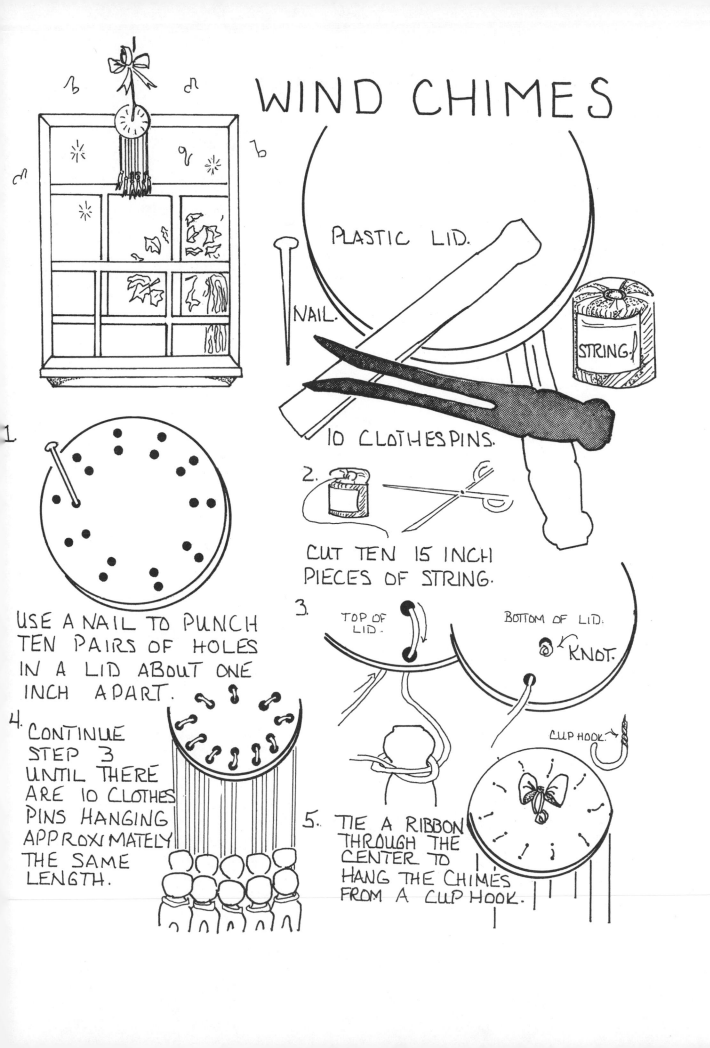

PLASTIC LID.

NAIL.

STRING.

10 CLOTHESPINS.

1. USE A NAIL TO PUNCH TEN PAIRS OF HOLES IN A LID ABOUT ONE INCH APART.

2. CUT TEN 15 INCH PIECES OF STRING.

3. TOP OF LID. BOTTOM OF LID. KNOT.

CUP HOOK.

4. CONTINUE STEP 3 UNTIL THERE ARE 10 CLOTHES PINS HANGING APPROXIMATELY THE SAME LENGTH.

5. TIE A RIBBON THROUGH THE CENTER TO HANG THE CHIMES FROM A CUP HOOK.

PAPER FLOWERS

Level of difficulty: *

MATERIALS: Colored tissue paper, scissors, floral wire cut in 16-inch lengths.

APPLICATIONS: These festive flowers brighten any room when put in a vase or taped to the wall. It is nice to give the flowers to nonambulatory friends on their birthdays or as get well wishes.

PREPARATION BEFORE CRAFT SESSION: Cut the pieces of tissue in half to make pieces approximately 15 inches by 20 inches. They do not have to be exact. Then stack two or three pieces of tissue in the same or varied colors and fold to make a paper fan. Tie each fan in the center with a piece of floral wire. Make dozens.

CRAFT SESSION: Separate the layers of tissue paper on both sides of the wire. The ruffled paper will now look like frilly flower petals.

PAPER FLOWERS

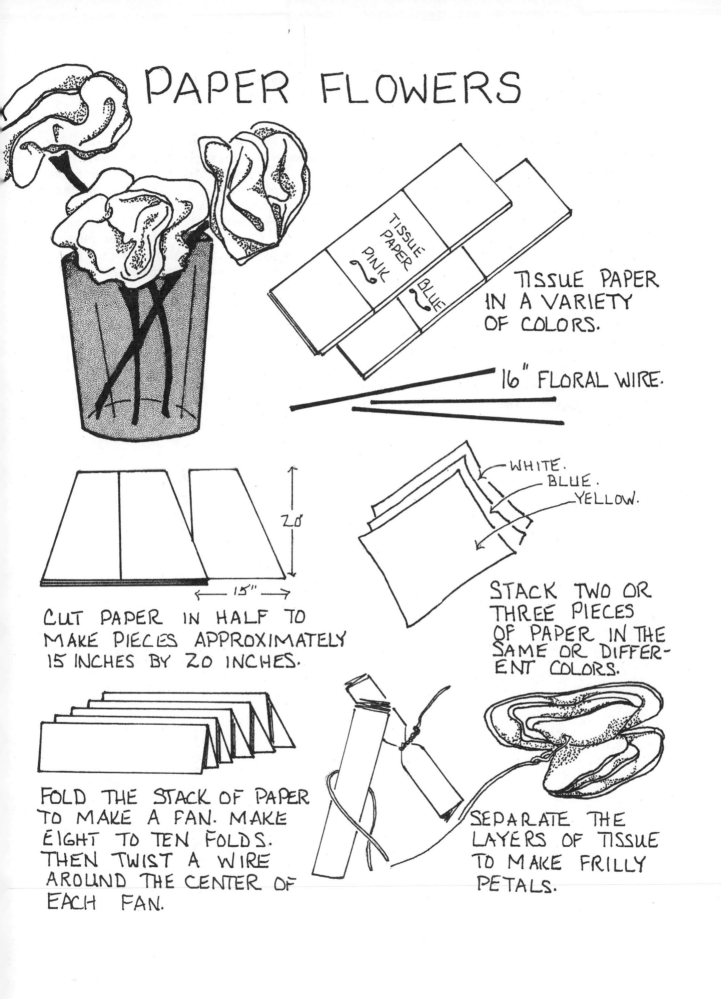

TISSUE PAPER PINK

BLUE

TISSUE PAPER IN A VARIETY OF COLORS.

16" FLORAL WIRE.

WHITE.
BLUE.
YELLOW.

20"

15"

CUT PAPER IN HALF TO MAKE PIECES APPROXIMATELY 15 INCHES BY 20 INCHES.

STACK TWO OR THREE PIECES OF PAPER IN THE SAME OR DIFFERENT COLORS.

FOLD THE STACK OF PAPER TO MAKE A FAN. MAKE EIGHT TO TEN FOLDS. THEN TWIST A WIRE AROUND THE CENTER OF EACH FAN.

SEPARATE THE LAYERS OF TISSUE TO MAKE FRILLY PETALS.

MOBILES

Level of difficulty: **—*****

MATERIALS: White drawing paper, black felt marking pen, wax paper, colored tissue paper, nylon thread, iron, 12-inch stick or dowel or wire from a coat hanger, glue stick, scissors, needle, thumbtacks.

APPLICATIONS: Mobiles have attracted the eyes of children and adults for centuries. These colorful butterflies shimmer with changing patterns when hung from a ceiling. Share the mobiles with nonambulatory patients.

PREPARATION BEFORE CRAFT SESSION: Using a black pen, trace five butterfly patterns on each piece of white drawing paper. Leave about 2 inches between each butterfly. Use glue stick to secure the papers to the table in front of each person. Then use the glue stick again to cover each piece of drawing paper with a piece of wax paper.

CRAFT SESSION: Arrange scraps of colored tissue paper on the wax paper to look like butterflies. The patterns on the drawing paper will help, but remember that the butterflies do not have to be perfect. Carefully place the other piece of wax paper over the tissue paper scraps. Press with a warm iron. Be sure no patients are near the warm iron or its cord.

This process will seal the designs between the wax papers. Cut out the butterflies leaving ¼-inch border of wax paper around each one. Using nylon thread and a needle to puncture the wax paper, tie five butterflies to each stick or wire. Tie one or two pieces of thread to the stick to hang the completed mobile from the ceiling with thumbtacks.

MOBILES

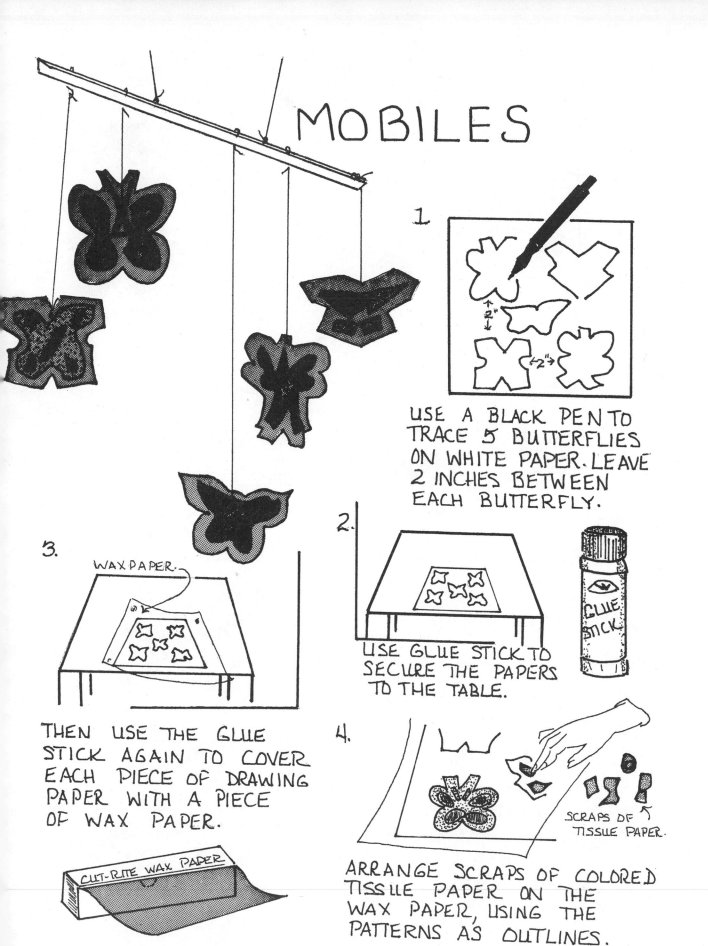

1

USE A BLACK PEN TO
TRACE 5 BUTTERFLIES
ON WHITE PAPER. LEAVE
2 INCHES BETWEEN
EACH BUTTERFLY.

2.

USE GLUE STICK TO
SECURE THE PAPERS
TO THE TABLE.

GLUE STICK

3.

WAX PAPER.

THEN USE THE GLUE
STICK AGAIN TO COVER
EACH PIECE OF DRAWING
PAPER WITH A PIECE
OF WAX PAPER.

CUT-RITE WAX PAPER

4.

SCRAPS OF
TISSUE PAPER.

ARRANGE SCRAPS OF COLORED
TISSUE PAPER ON THE
WAX PAPER, USING THE
PATTERNS AS OUTLINES.

MOBILES

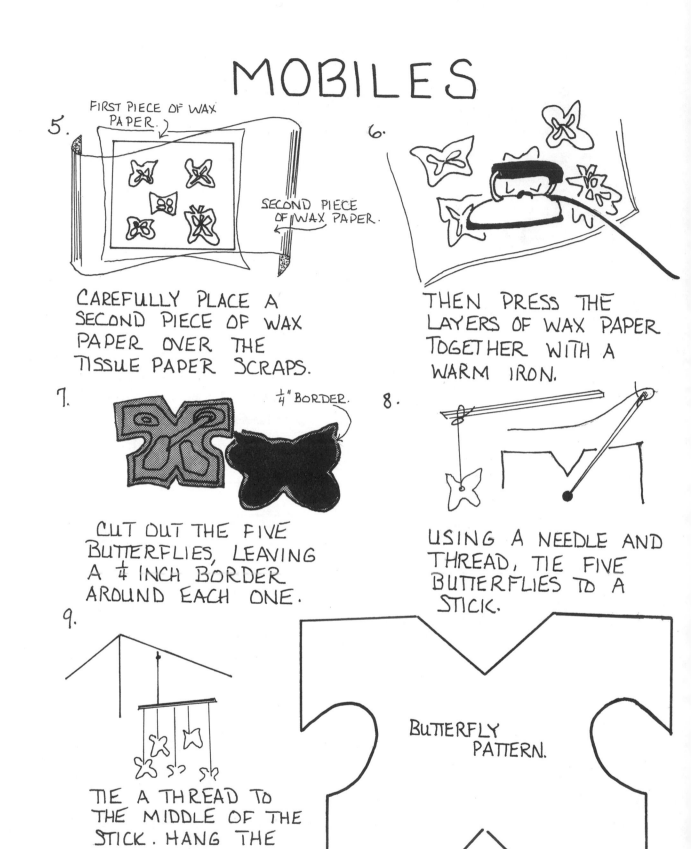

5. FIRST PIECE OF WAX PAPER.

SECOND PIECE OF WAX PAPER.

CAREFULLY PLACE A SECOND PIECE OF WAX PAPER OVER THE TISSUE PAPER SCRAPS.

6. THEN PRESS THE LAYERS OF WAX PAPER TOGETHER WITH A WARM IRON.

7. $\frac{1}{4}$" BORDER.

CUT OUT THE FIVE BUTTERFLIES, LEAVING A $\frac{1}{4}$ INCH BORDER AROUND EACH ONE.

8. USING A NEEDLE AND THREAD, TIE FIVE BUTTERFLIES TO A STICK.

9. TIE A THREAD TO THE MIDDLE OF THE STICK. HANG THE MOBILE FROM THE CEILING WITH A TACK.

BUTTERFLY PATTERN.

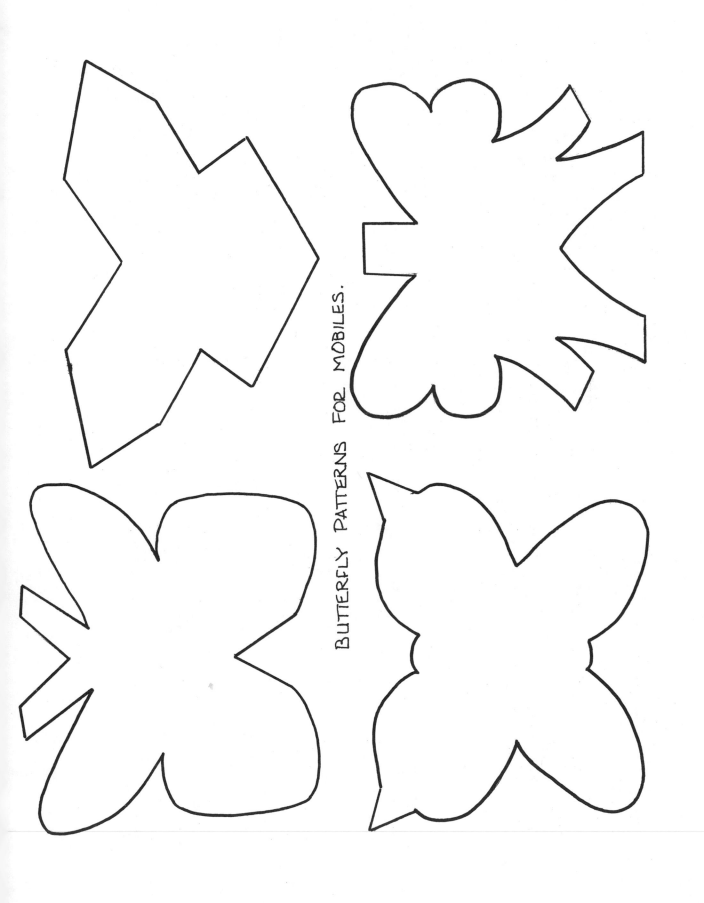

BUTTERFLY PATTERNS FOR MOBILES.

SPRING PLANT-IN

Level of difficulty: **–*****

MATERIALS: Plastic or clay flower pots, contact paper, scissors, newspaper, water, potting soil, seeds.

APPLICATIONS: In the springtime, thoughts turn to nature. Let each person who is able, plant and decorate a flower pot. Then put all the pots together along the walkways of your nursing home or in a central patio. Let ambulatory patients be in charge of watering the pots. Everyone can enjoy the blossoms. Nurseries will be happy to donate old pots, or use gallon size plastic food containers with holes punched in the bottoms for drainage.

PREPARATION BEFORE CRAFT SESSION: None.

CRAFT SESSION: Cut flowers out of contact paper. Peel off the backing, and stick the contact paper flowers on the pots for decoration. Spread newspapers to catch dirt. Fill the pots with soil. Plant the seeds and water them. Place the pots outside in an easy-to-see location.

SPRING PLANT-IN

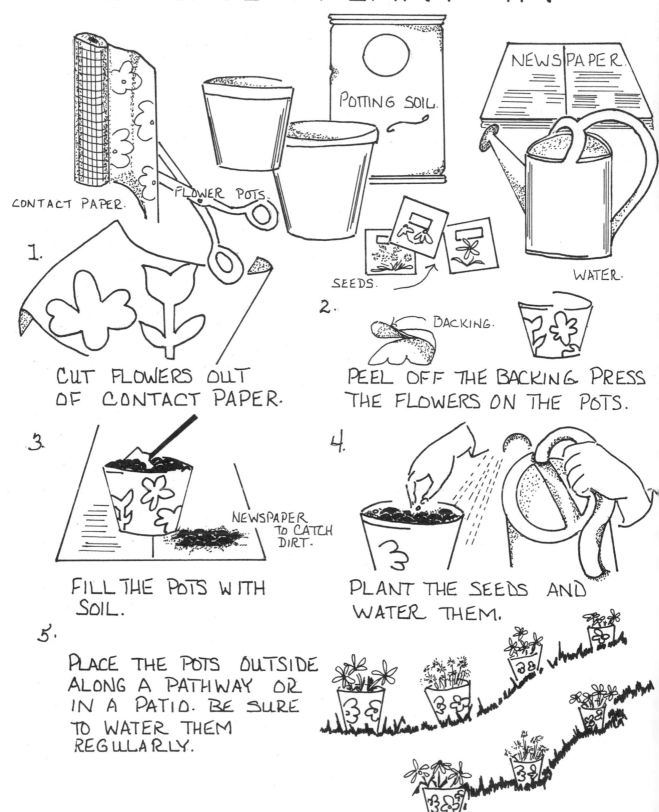

CONTACT PAPER.

FLOWER POTS.

POTTING SOIL.

NEWSPAPER.

SEEDS.

WATER.

1. CUT FLOWERS OUT OF CONTACT PAPER.

2. BACKING.

PEEL OFF THE BACKING PRESS THE FLOWERS ON THE POTS.

3. NEWSPAPER TO CATCH DIRT.

FILL THE POTS WITH SOIL.

4. PLANT THE SEEDS AND WATER THEM.

5. PLACE THE POTS OUTSIDE ALONG A PATHWAY OR IN A PATIO. BE SURE TO WATER THEM REGULARLY.

PATTERNS FOR FLOWER CUT-OUTS

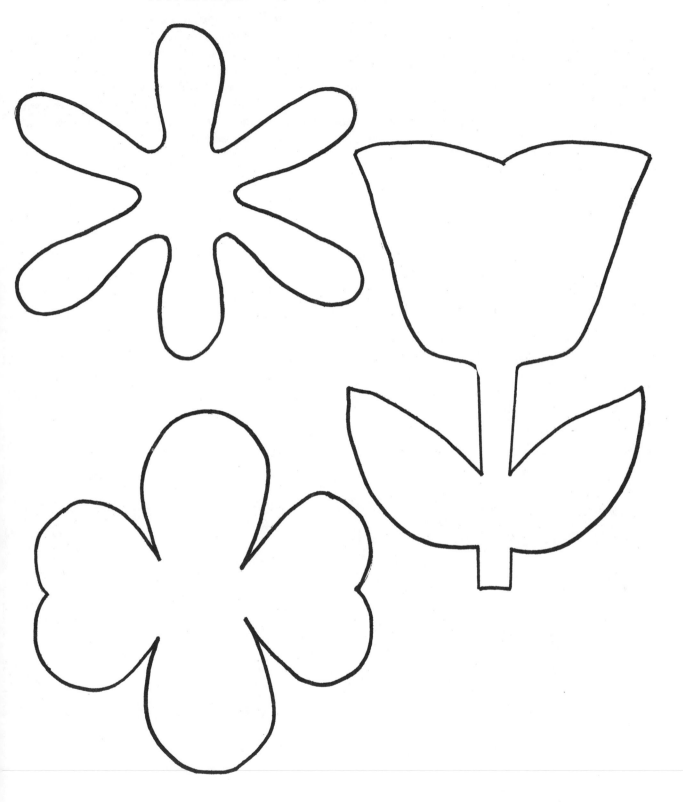

GREETING CARD HOLDERS

Level of difficulty: **

MATERIALS: 46-ounce juice cans, yarn, scissors.

APPLICATIONS: The card holder is nice to hold get-well cards on a dresser or night stand. Use red and green yarn for Christmas or pink and blue yarn for a baby shower gift.

PREPARATION BEFORE CRAFT SESSION: Wash cans and cut out both ends of each can. Loop the yarn through the can and tie a knot to secure the yarn.

CRAFT SESSION: Have each person wind the yarn through the can over and over again until the entire can is covered with yarn. It is best to pull the yarn as tight as possible. When the can is covered with yarn, help each person cut and knot the yarn on the inside of the can. The holder is now ready to have cards inserted.

GREETING CARD HOLDERS

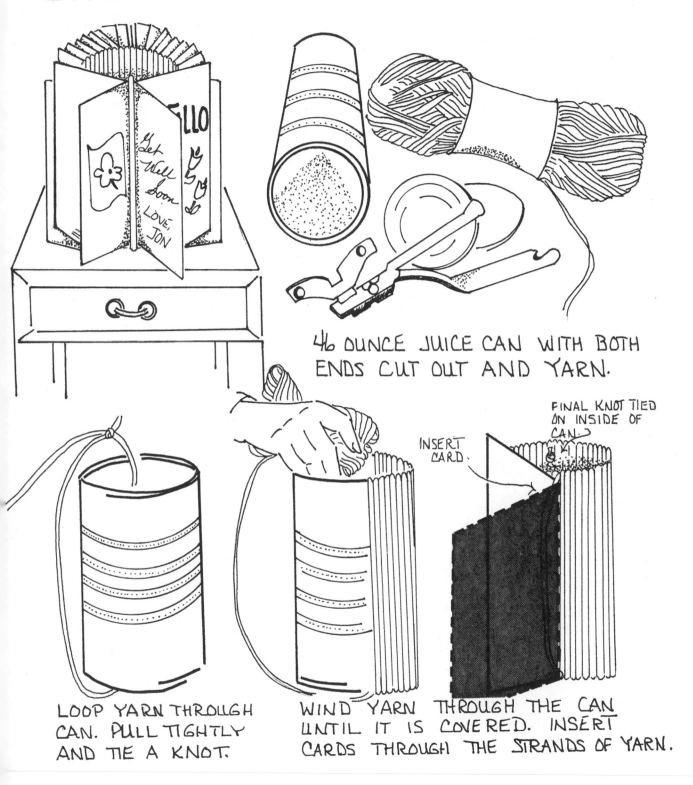

46 OUNCE JUICE CAN WITH BOTH ENDS CUT OUT AND YARN.

FINAL KNOT TIED ON INSIDE OF CAN.

INSERT CARD.

LOOP YARN THROUGH CAN. PULL TIGHTLY AND TIE A KNOT.

WIND YARN THROUGH THE CAN UNTIL IT IS COVERED. INSERT CARDS THROUGH THE STRANDS OF YARN.

BEDSIDE RACKS

Level of difficulty: *

MATERIALS: 46 ounce juice cans, fabric, pinking shears, glue, ribbon.

APPLICATIONS: The bedside rack is nice to hold magazines or tissues. Tie the racks with the ribbon to headboards or the inside of bed rails for patients who cannot reach their night stands.

PREPARATION BEFORE CRAFT SESSION: Wash cans and cut out both ends of each can. Cut ribbon into 36-inch lengths. Cut fabric with pinking shears into pieces 7¼ inches by 13½ inches.

CRAFT SESSION: Glue the fabric to the can. Loop the ribbon through the can and tie a bow.

BEDSIDE RACKS

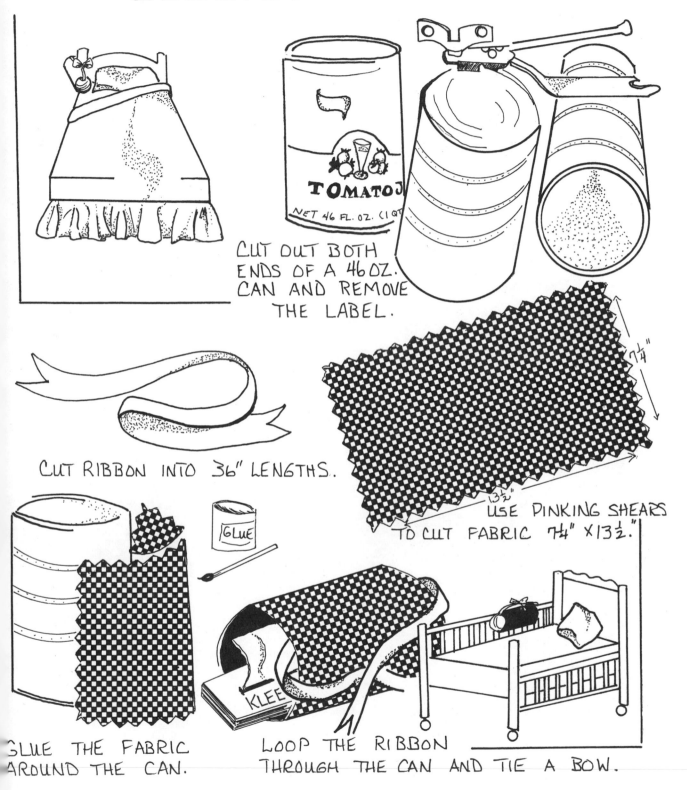

CUT OUT BOTH ENDS OF A 46 OZ. CAN AND REMOVE THE LABEL.

TOMATO

NET 46 FL. OZ. (1 QT)

CUT RIBBON INTO 36" LENGTHS.

USE PINKING SHEARS TO CUT FABRIC 7¼" X 13½."

GLUE

KLEE

GLUE THE FABRIC AROUND THE CAN.

LOOP THE RIBBON THROUGH THE CAN AND TIE A BOW.

EASTER CENTERPIECES

Level of difficulty: *—***

MATERIALS: Yellow construction paper, scissors, glue, felt marking pens or crayons, paper plates, small candy eggs, cellophane grass, glue stick.

APPLICATIONS: These easy-to-make holiday centerpieces are nice to brighten a bleak room of a nonambulatory patient. Also, make many centerpieces and use them to decorate the dining-hall tables of your home or institution. Be careful that candy eggs are not in the reach of diabetics. You may prefer to substitute plastic eggs.

PREPARATION BEFORE CRAFT SESSION: Trace two patterns of each figure and cut them out of yellow construction paper. Note the illustration. Using glue stick, secure two patterns of each figure facing each other in front of each person. There will be a total of six cutouts for each centerpiece.

CRAFT SESSION: Color the cutouts with pens or crayons. Spread glue near the top on the back of each figure, and paste them together; the bottom part is not pasted, as it spreads apart. Fold the bases outward, each side in an opposite direction. Then spread glue on the bottom of the base of each figure, and paste the three figures on a paper plate. Arrange cellophane grass and eggs between and around the figures.

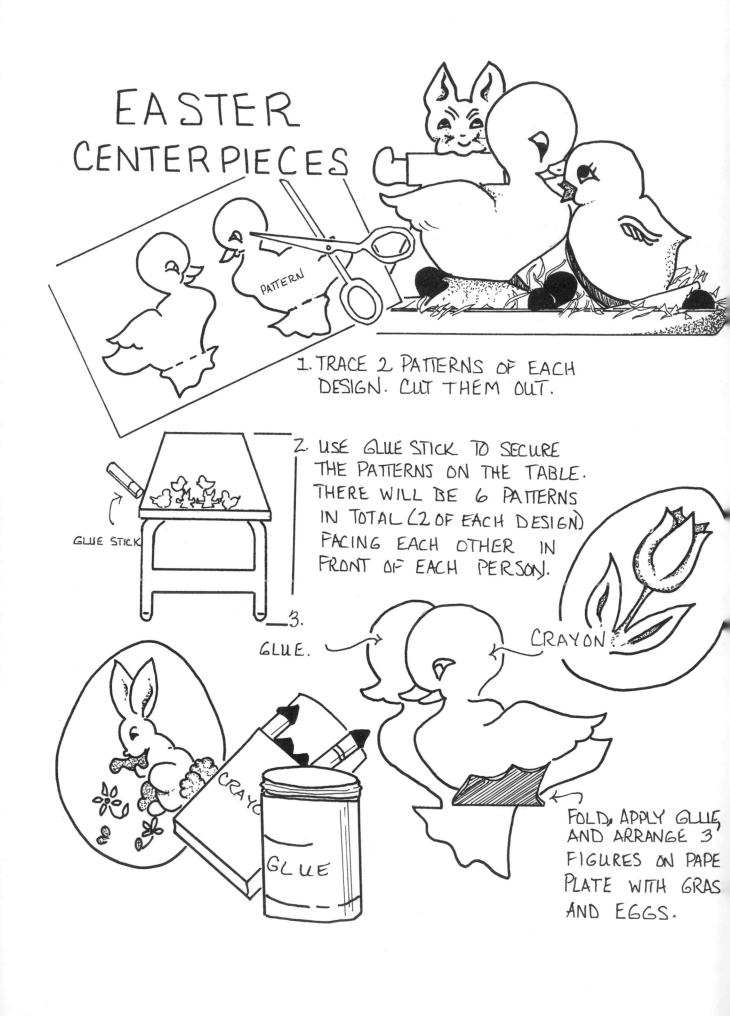

EASTER CENTERPIECES

PATTERN

1. TRACE 2 PATTERNS OF EACH DESIGN. CUT THEM OUT.

GLUE STICK

2. USE GLUE STICK TO SECURE THE PATTERNS ON THE TABLE. THERE WILL BE 6 PATTERNS IN TOTAL (2 OF EACH DESIGN) FACING EACH OTHER IN FRONT OF EACH PERSON.

3. GLUE.

CRAYON

CRAYON

GLUE

FOLD, APPLY GLUE, AND ARRANGE 3 FIGURES ON PAPE PLATE WITH GRAS AND EGGS.

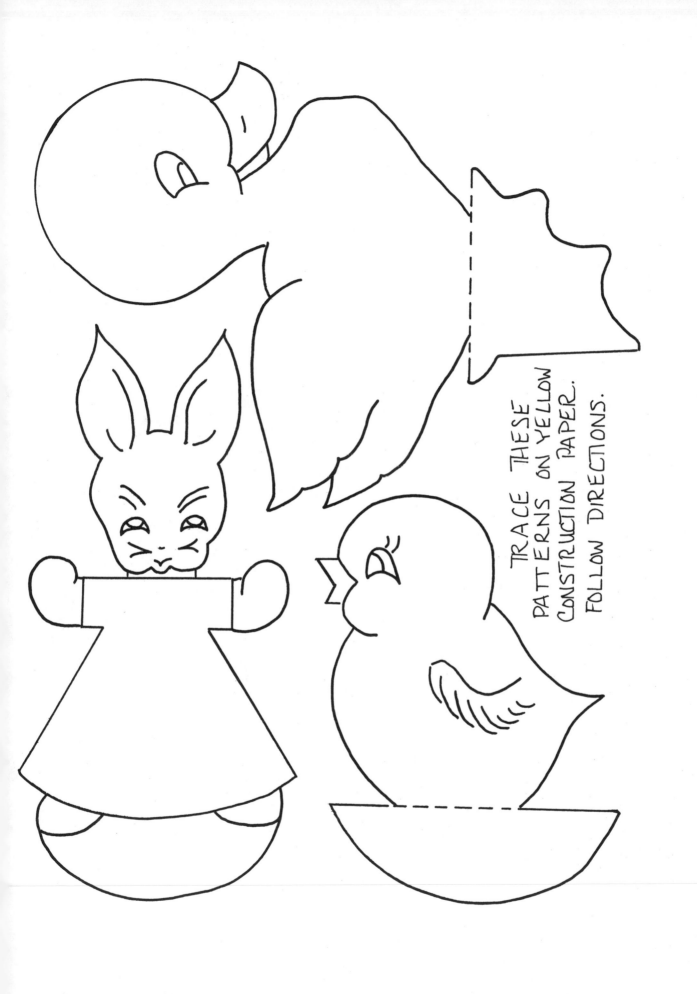

TRACE THESE
PATTERNS ON YELLOW
CONSTRUCTION PAPER.
FOLLOW DIRECTIONS.

CHAPTER FIVE

Craft Projects to Give to Family Members

SOUP RECIPES

Level of difficulty: **—*****

MATERIALS: Empty soup can with label, plastic vegetables or flowers, floral clay or Styrofoam®, plastic fork, 5 x 7 file card, recipes, black felt marking pens.

APPLICATIONS: Most people have a favorite recipe to share with their families. This is a pretty reminder of "Aunt Esther's" wisdom and also makes a unique and special kitchen shower gift.

PREPARATION BEFORE CRAFT SESSION: Wash soup cans carefully taking care not to soil the label, which remains on the can. Bring a recipe for each type soup can you have for those people who cannot remember or do not have their own recipes (example: Split pea, vegetable, onion, chicken).

CRAFT SESSION: Fill the can with clay or Styrofoam. Using the plastic vegetables and flowers, make an attractive arrangement with the can as the vase. Insert a plastic fork upside down into the arrangement. Help each person write down his favorite recipe on a file card. Be sure to include signatures or names. Then insert the card through the tines of the fork.

SOUP RECIPES

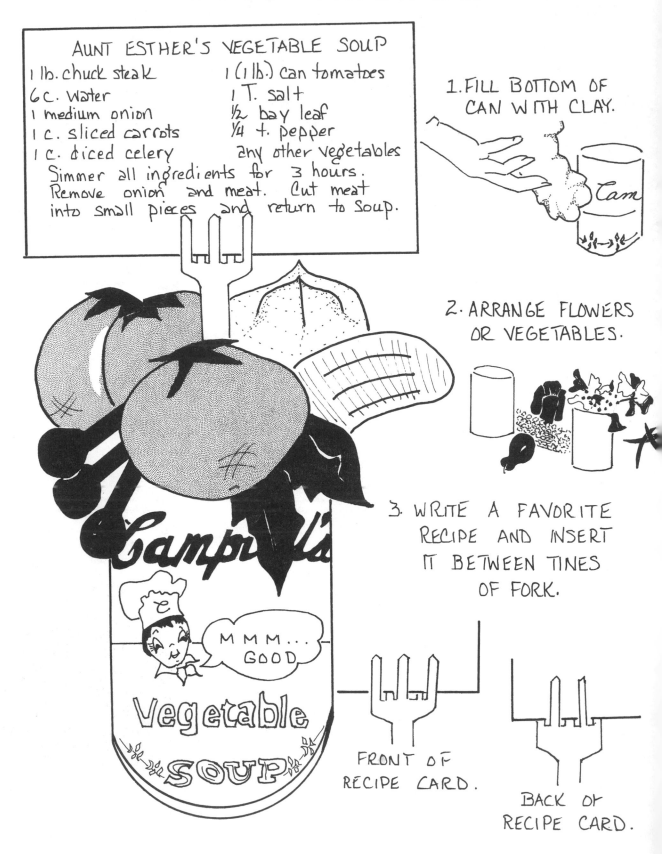

AUNT ESTHER'S VEGETABLE SOUP

1 lb. chuck steak	1 (1 lb.) can tomatoes
6 c. water	1 T. salt
1 medium onion	½ bay leaf
1 c. sliced carrots	¼ t. pepper
1 c. diced celery	any other vegetables

Simmer all ingredients for 3 hours. Remove onion and meat. Cut meat into small pieces and return to soup.

1. FILL BOTTOM OF CAN WITH CLAY.

2. ARRANGE FLOWERS OR VEGETABLES.

3. WRITE A FAVORITE RECIPE AND INSERT IT BETWEEN TINES OF FORK.

FRONT OF RECIPE CARD.

BACK OF RECIPE CARD.

EXTRA RECIPES

SPLIT PEA SOUP

1 large ham bone
1 lb. split peas
3 quarts water
1 white onion
1/2 carrot (diced)

Salt, red & white pepper
6 slices bacon (optional)
2 hard cooked eggs (optional)

Boil peas and ham until peas dissolve. Add seasoning and simmer 2½ hours. Put soup through sieve. Replace ham bits in soup. Sprinkle bacon crumbs & chopped egg over each serving.

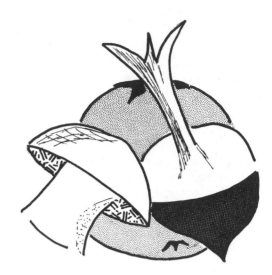

TOMATO SOUP

2 c. tomato juice
1 rib celery
1/4 medium green pepper
2 medium carrots
1 medium tomato
1/2 cucumber

salt
tobasco
pepper
worcestershire sauce
1/2 sliced lime or lemon

Chop all vegetables. Add seasoning to taste. Chill thoroughly. Serve in bowl with slice of lime.

CHICKEN SOUP

6 sprigs parsley
1/4 t. thyme
1 T. salt
1/4 t. pepper

3 lb. hen
3 quarts water
3 c. chopped celery
1 large onion
2 carrots, diced

Simmer all ingredients 3 hours. Pour through a sieve. Save chicken for salads. Rice or noodles may then be cooked in the broth.

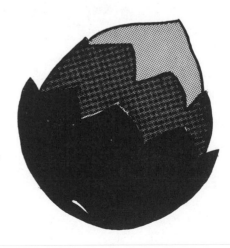

LUNCH BAGS

Level of difficulty: *—**

MATERIALS: Colored art paper, lunch bags, scissors, craft glue, brush.

APPLICATIONS: Children adore decorated lunch bags for school or camp. Patients can even personalize the bags with their grandchildren's names worked into the design. These bags are almost too easy to make, but they are clever and eye-catching. They are just the project to interest an otherwise reluctant person. I especially like to cut out the designs nonchalantly while carrying on a conversation with my patient. He would become intrigued and was more open to mutual participation in a project the next time I asked.

PREPARATION BEFORE CRAFT SESSION: Cut designs out of colored paper. Curl eyelashes, whiskers, and hair by winding the paper tightly around the end of a brush and then releasing it. Be creative or copy the patterns in the illustrations.

CRAFT SESSION: Apply glue to the cutouts. Press in place. Cut out names and "lunch" or "bag" out of paper, and glue these on, too.

LUNCH BAGS

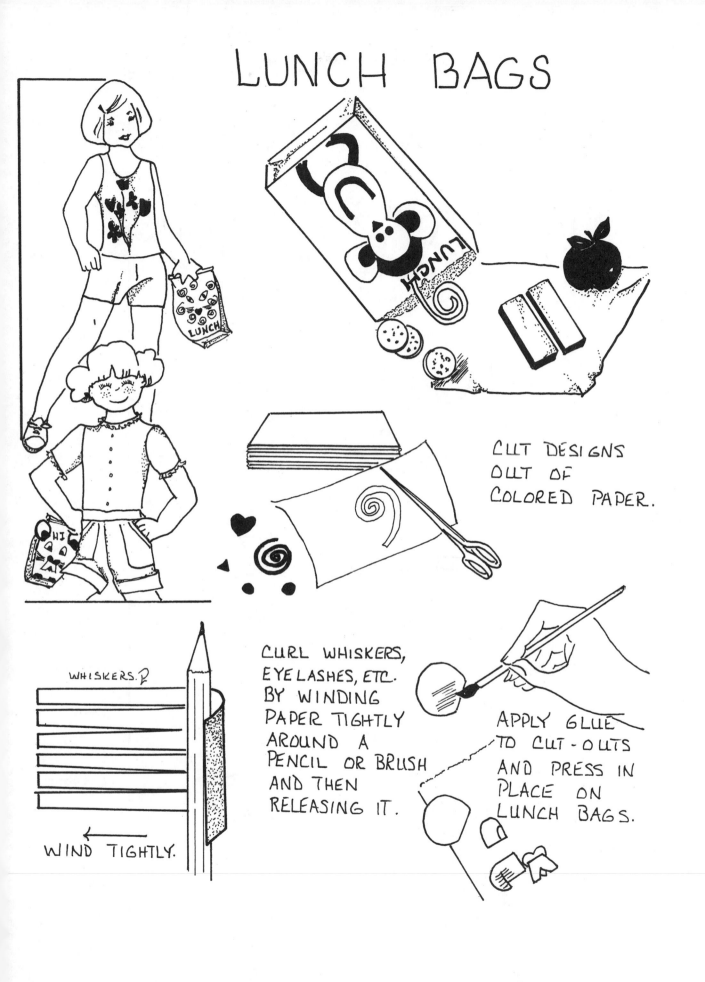

CUT DESIGNS OUT OF COLORED PAPER.

CURL WHISKERS, EYELASHES, ETC. BY WINDING PAPER TIGHTLY AROUND A PENCIL OR BRUSH AND THEN RELEASING IT.

APPLY GLUE TO CUT-OUTS AND PRESS IN PLACE ON LUNCH BAGS.

WHISKERS.

WIND TIGHTLY.

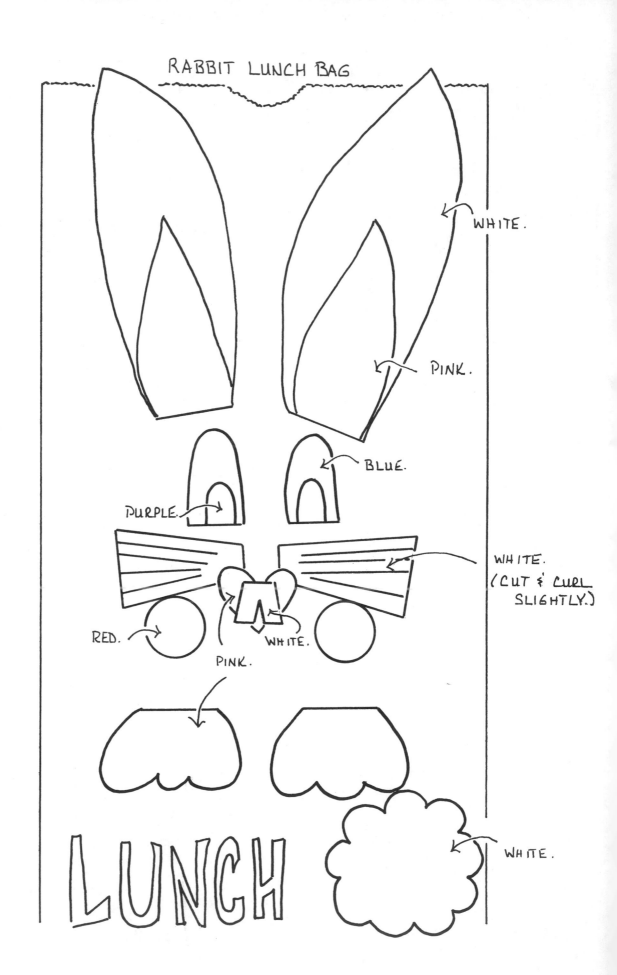

RABBIT LUNCH BAG

WHITE.

PINK.

BLUE.

PURPLE.

WHITE.
(CUT & CURL
SLIGHTLY.)

RED.

WHITE.

PINK.

LUNCH

WHITE.

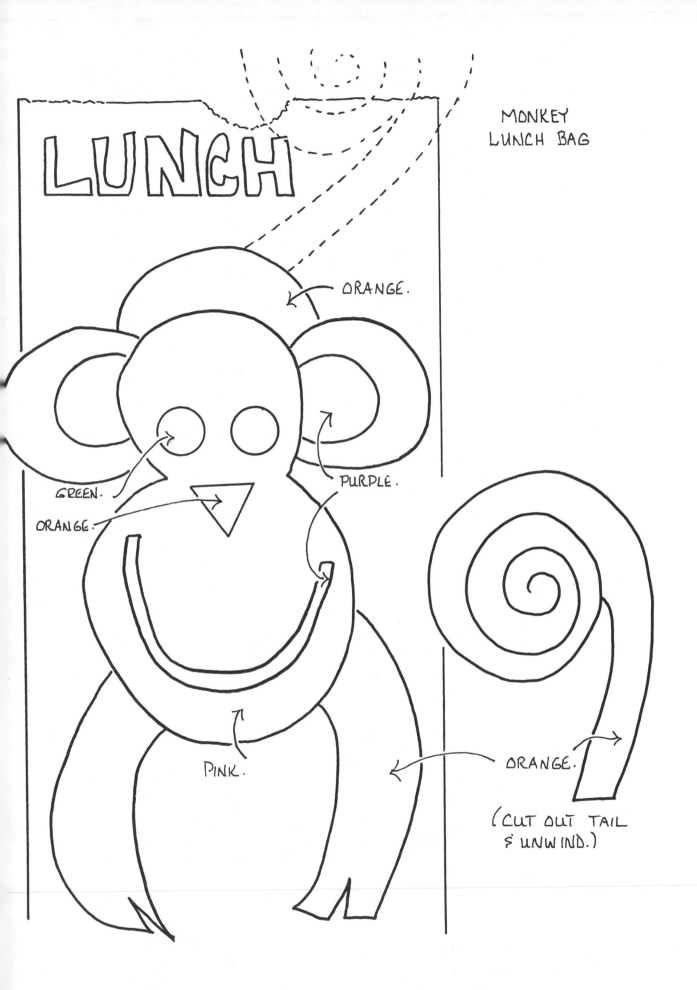

MONKEY
LUNCH BAG

LUNCH

ORANGE.

GREEN.

ORANGE.

PURPLE.

PINK.

ORANGE.

(CUT OUT TAIL
& UNWIND.)

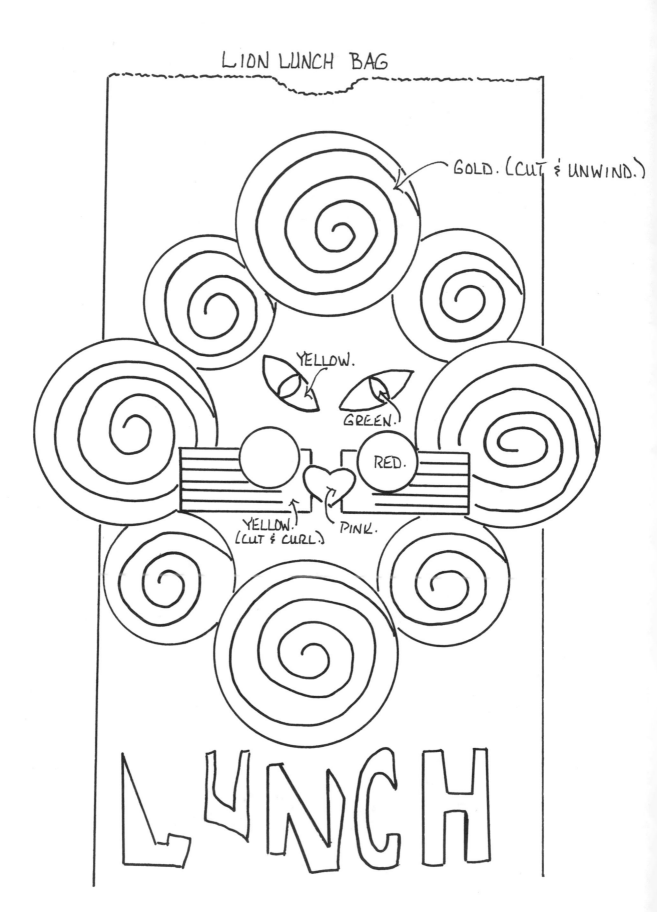

RED RIDING HOOD LUNCH BAG

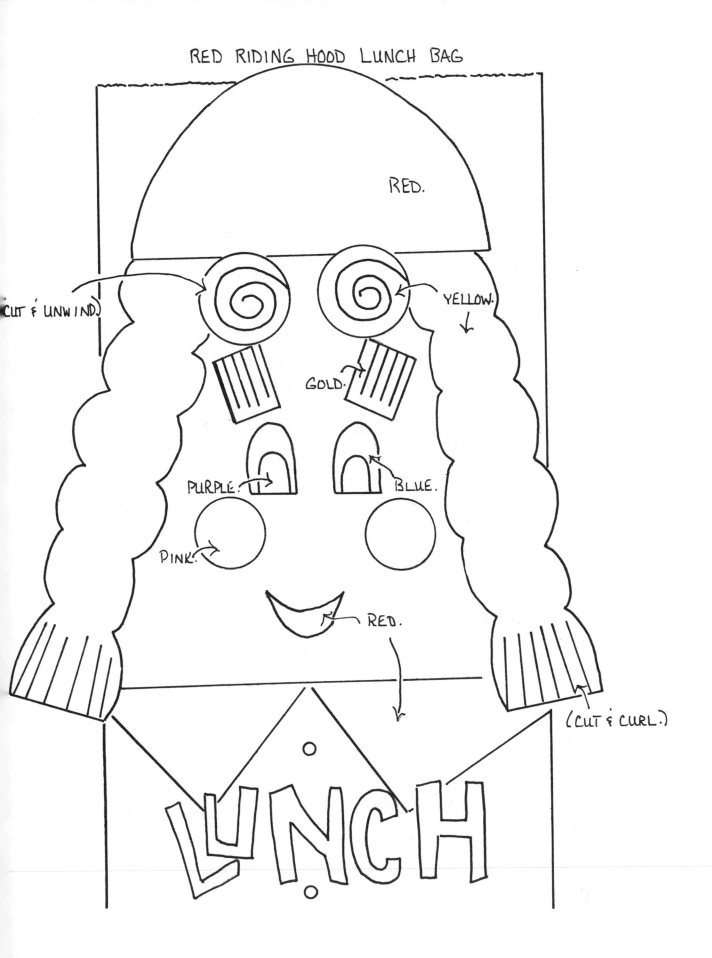

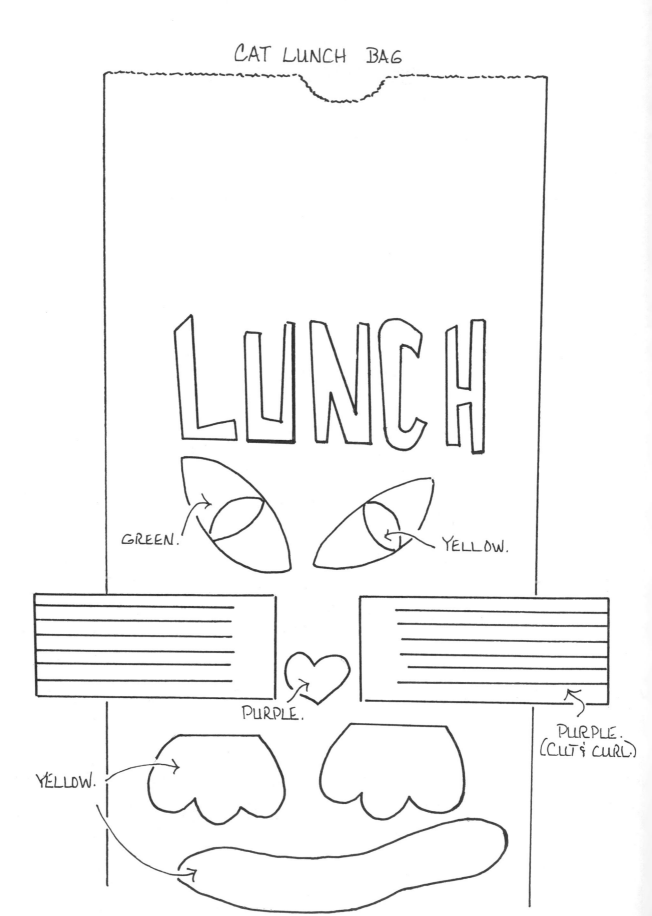

CAT LUNCH BAG

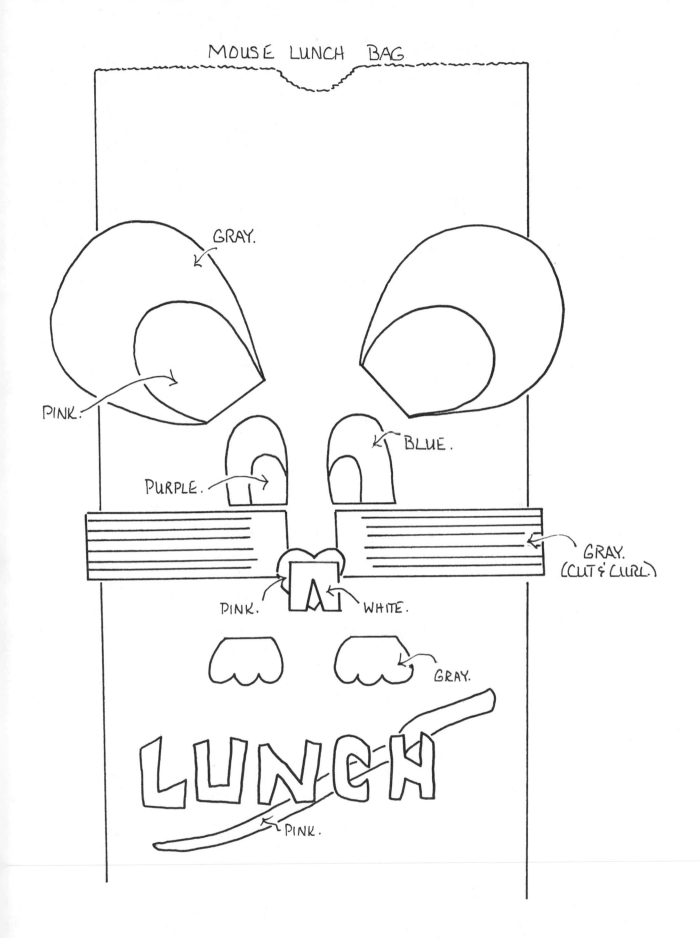

CANDY BOWL

Level of difficulty: *—**

MATERIALS: Empty margarine tubs, 27 round-headed clothespins for each bowl, wood stain (optional).

APPLICATIONS: It is hard to believe this candy bowl was once a margarine tub and clothespins. Fill it with mints before giving it away for an extra nice gift.

PREPARATION BEFORE CRAFT SESSION: If you like, stain the clothespins and allow them to dry.

CRAFT SESSION: Simply put the clothespins over the edge of the tub and push them close together. Fill the bowl with candy for a clothespin studded candy bowl.

CANDY BOWL

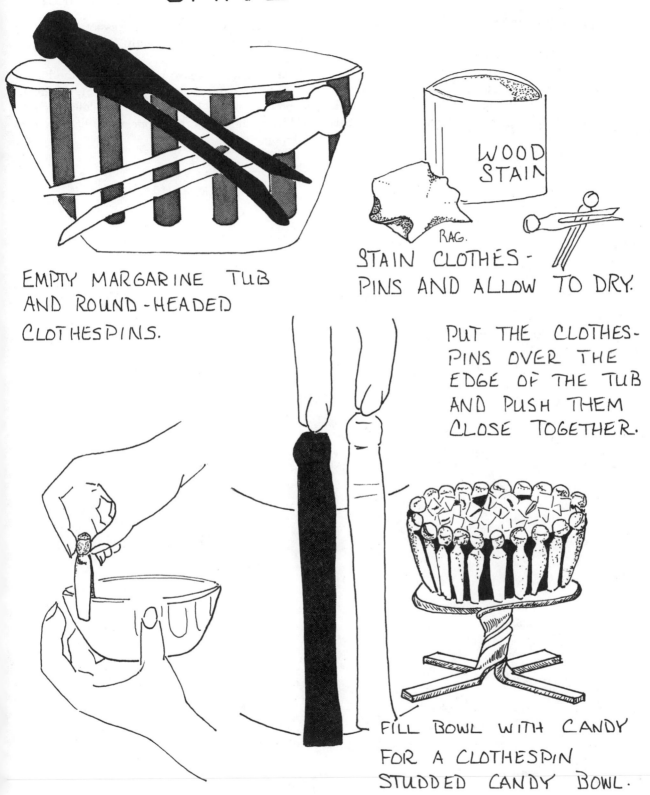

EMPTY MARGARINE TUB AND ROUND-HEADED CLOTHESPINS.

WOOD STAIN

RAG.

STAIN CLOTHES-PINS AND ALLOW TO DRY.

PUT THE CLOTHES-PINS OVER THE EDGE OF THE TUB AND PUSH THEM CLOSE TOGETHER.

FILL BOWL WITH CANDY FOR A CLOTHESPIN STUDDED CANDY BOWL.

Level of difficulty: **—***

MATERIALS: Empty plastic produce baskets, ribbon, 1-inch thick Styrofoam, lollipops, knife.

APPLICATIONS: A whole basket of lollipops appeals to every child. If you do not have a special child in mind for your basket, donate it to a local hospital.

LOLLIPOP BASKETS

PREPARATION BEFORE CRAFT SESSION: Cut the Styrofoam in squares to exactly fit the bottom of a basket.

CRAFT SESSION: Weave ribbon around the basket and tie it in a bow. Put a piece of Styrofoam in the bottom of the basket. Poke the lollipops into the Styrofoam. Be sure no one with diabetes eats a lollipop.

LOLLIPOP BASKETS

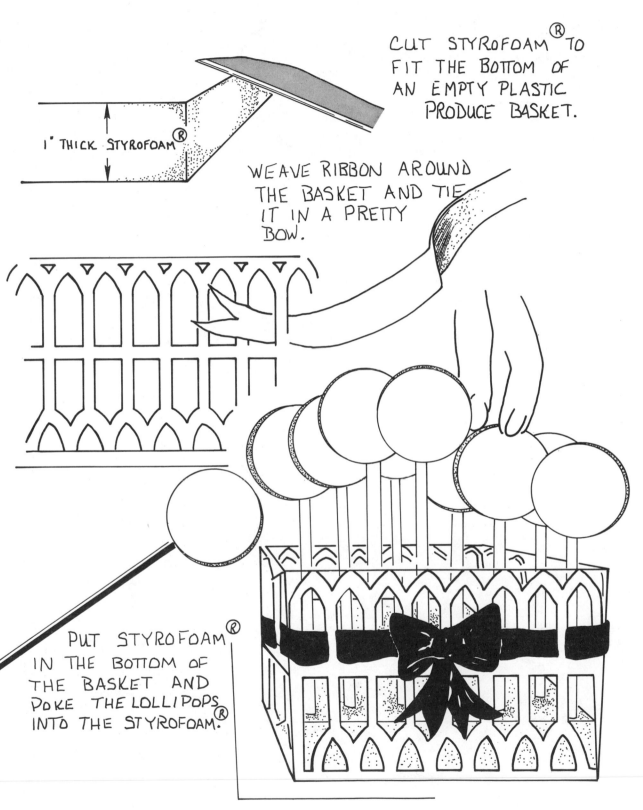

1" THICK STYROFOAM®

CUT STYROFOAM® TO FIT THE BOTTOM OF AN EMPTY PLASTIC PRODUCE BASKET.

WEAVE RIBBON AROUND THE BASKET AND TIE IT IN A PRETTY BOW.

PUT STYROFOAM® IN THE BOTTOM OF THE BASKET AND POKE THE LOLLIPOPS INTO THE STYROFOAM.®

TOY SNAKES

Level of difficulty: ***—*****

MATERIALS: Fabric, toilet paper tubes, buttons, red ribbon or bias binding, knee socks or stockings, paper towels, glue, pinking shears (Stapler and staples, optional).

APPLICATIONS: The wiggly toy snakes appeal to young grandchildren. They also make a nice contribution to a local church or school bazaar or the pediatric ward of a hospital.

PREPARATION BEFORE CRAFT SESSION: Cut red forked tongues about 3 inches in length. Cut fabric (calico is especially appealing) into pieces 5 inches by 6 inches.

CRAFT SESSION: Cover five tubes with cloth for each snake. The simplest way is to paint a stripe of glue down a tube. Secure the cloth. Then wind the cloth around the tube and glue the overlap. Stuff paper towels into the toe of a sock to form the head. String the tubes onto the sock, knotting several socks together for added length. When the last one is on, tie a large knot in the tail end. Then glue on two buttons for the eyes and the ribbon for the tongue. The end knot may be stapled to the end tube for added security.

TOY SNAKES

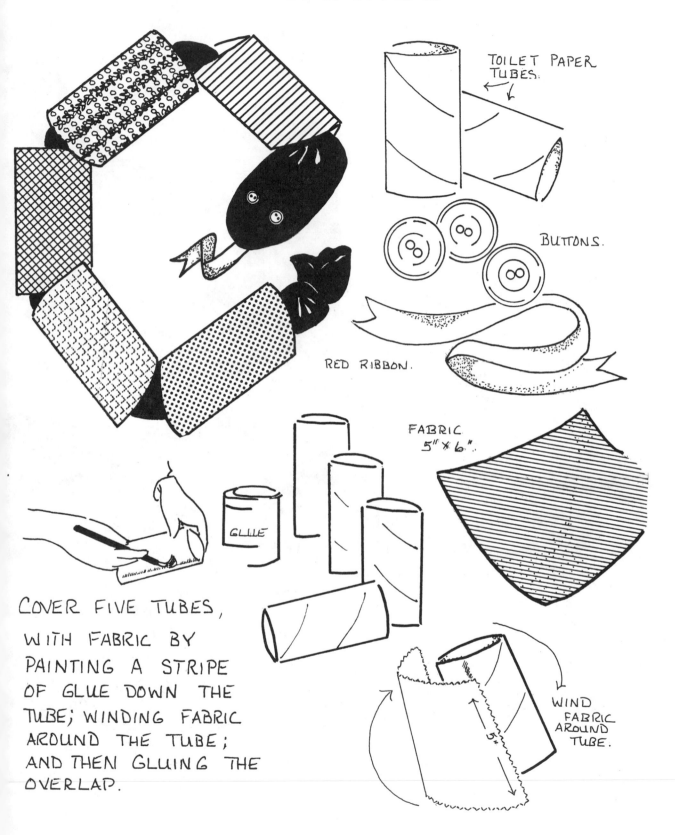

TOILET PAPER TUBES.

BUTTONS.

RED RIBBON.

FABRIC 5" × 6"

GLUE

COVER FIVE TUBES, WITH FABRIC BY PAINTING A STRIPE OF GLUE DOWN THE TUBE; WINDING FABRIC AROUND THE TUBE; AND THEN GLUING THE OVERLAP.

5"

WIND FABRIC AROUND TUBE.

TOY SNAKES

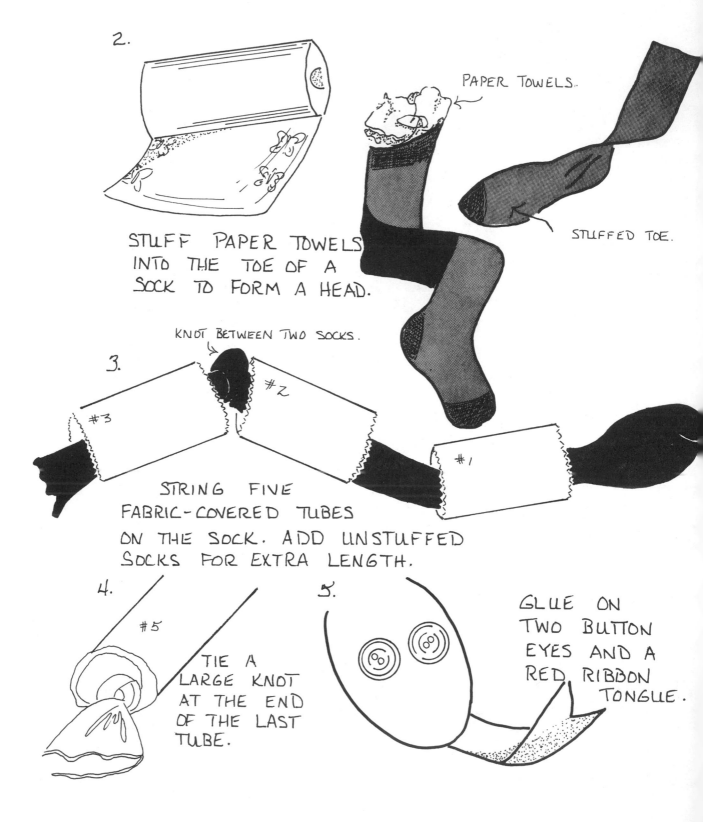

2.

STUFF PAPER TOWELS INTO THE TOE OF A SOCK TO FORM A HEAD.

PAPER TOWELS.

STUFFED TOE.

KNOT BETWEEN TWO SOCKS.

3.

#3

#2

#1

STRING FIVE FABRIC-COVERED TUBES ON THE SOCK. ADD UNSTUFFED SOCKS FOR EXTRA LENGTH.

4.

#5

TIE A LARGE KNOT AT THE END OF THE LAST TUBE.

5.

GLUE ON TWO BUTTON EYES AND A RED RIBBON TONGUE.

PATTERNS FOR TOY SNAKE

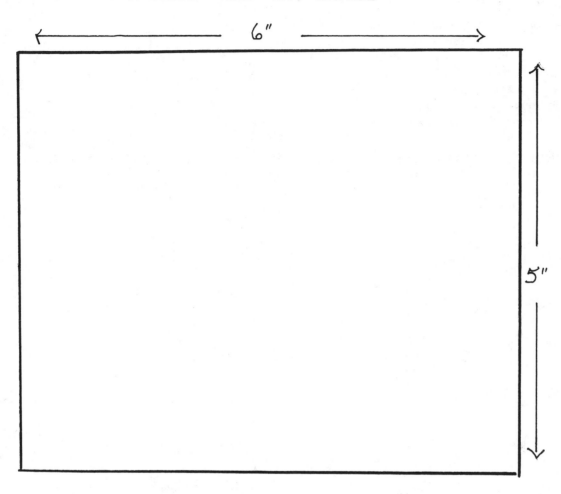

6"

5"

USE PINKING SHEARS TO CUT FIVE
PIECES OF FABRIC FOR EACH SNAKE.

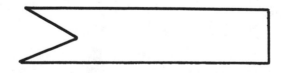

CUT ONE TONGUE PER SNAKE.

EASTER EGGS

Level of difficulty: * — * * * * *

MATERIALS: Eggs, needle, felt marking pens in a variety of colors, empty egg cartons, cellophane grass, paper bowls or baskets of any sort (example: empty plastic produce baskets).

APPLICATIONS: Personalized Easter eggs are special to family members; and if stored carefully, they stay pretty for years to display annually.

PREPARATION BEFORE CRAFT SESSION: Separate each egg section from a carton to serve as egg-holders for feeble hands that might otherwise crack a blown egg. Then blow eggs. To do this, begin by shaking the egg. Use a needle to make a hole at one end of the egg and another one a bit larger at the other end. Blow gently into the smaller hole until the yolk and white are completely out. Wash the shell and stand it on end to dry. (You can use the eggs for baking . . . just keep an accurate count.)

CRAFT SESSION: Put a blown egg in an egg carton section and let each person decorate in his own creative way. Traditional Easter bunnies and flowers are nice, but so are zig zags and colorful *scribbling*. Assemble half a dozen eggs on the cellophane grass in bowls or baskets.

EASTER EGGS

1.

USE A NEEDLE TO MAKE A HOLE AT EACH END OF AN EGG.

2.

BLOW THE EGG INTO A BOWL AND RINSE OUT THE EMPTY SHELL.

3.

BREAK CARTON INTO 12 SECTIONS.

PUT A BLOWN EGG IN AN EMPTY EGG CARTON SECTION. DECORATE THE EGG WITH FELT PENS.

4.

PUT EGGS IN BASKET OR BOWL WITH CELLOPHANE GRASS.

SAVINGS BANKS

Level of difficulty: *—***

MATERIALS: Empty pop-top soda cans, plain art paper, glue stick, craft glue, black felt marking pen, crayons, scissors, ric rac or ribbon, small paint brush, gummed labels (3 inch x 3 inch).

APPLICATIONS: Grandchildren especially like personalized little banks with their names on the outside and a couple of pennies that jingle on the inside. The banks are also nice to save a few coins for your favorite charity.

PREPARATION BEFORE CRAFT SESSION: Cut plain art paper to fit around pop-top soda cans (4½ inch x 8¼ inch). Trace patterns on the paper with a black felt pen. Using glue stick, secure the paper to the table in front of each person.

CRAFT SESSION: Have each person color the patterns with crayon. Using a paint brush, spread craft glue on the can and attach the colored pattern. Glue a trim of ric rac or ribbon on the top and bottom of the can. Then help each person design and write his own personalized label for the can. Be sure he signs his name. Attach the label to the can.

SAVINGS BANKS

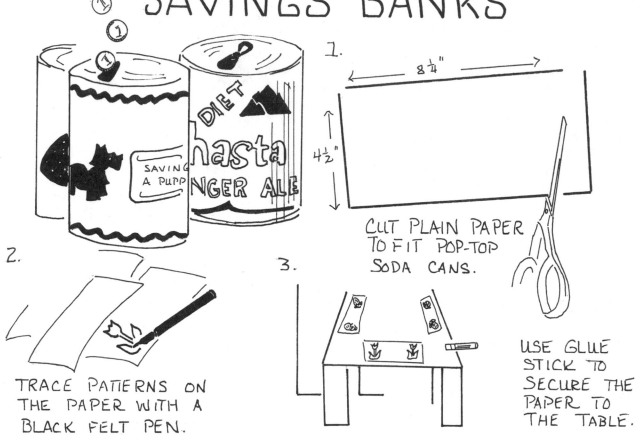

1. 8¼"   4½"

CUT PLAIN PAPER
TO FIT POP-TOP
SODA CANS.

2.

TRACE PATTERNS ON
THE PAPER WITH A
BLACK FELT PEN.

3.

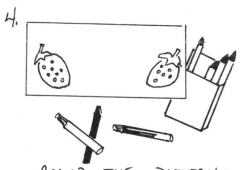

USE GLUE
STICK TO
SECURE THE
PAPER TO
THE TABLE.

4.

COLOR THE PATTERNS
WITH CRAYONS OR
FELT PENS.

5.

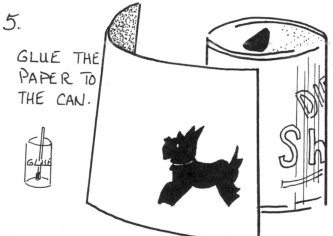

GLUE THE
PAPER TO
THE CAN.

GLUE

6.

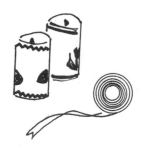

TRIM THE
TOP AND
BOTTOM EDGES
WITH RIC RAC
OR RIBBON.

7.

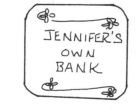

JENNIFER'S
OWN
BANK

ATTACH A
GUMMED LABEL
WITH A LITTLE
SAYING ON IT.

PATTERNS FOR SAVINGS BANKS

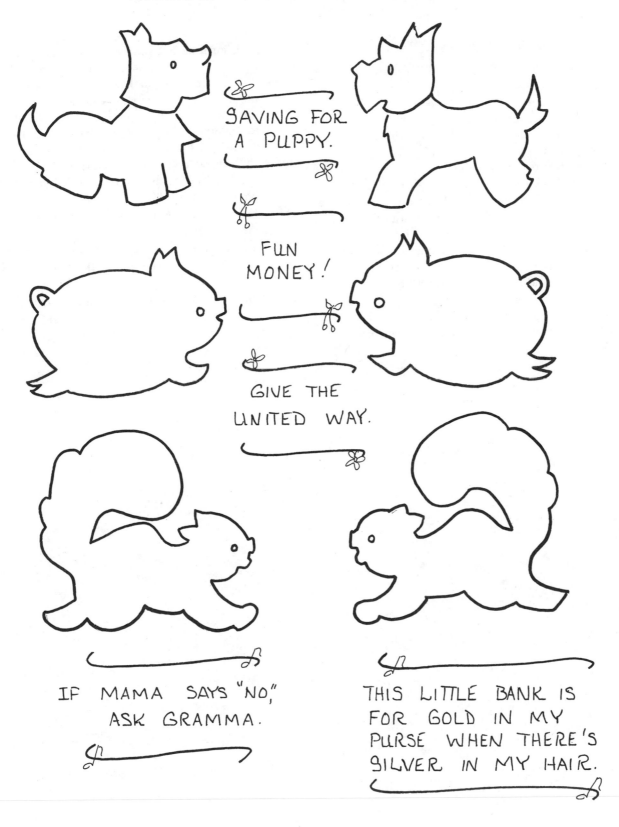

SAVING FOR A PUPPY.

FUN MONEY!

GIVE THE UNITED WAY.

IF MAMA SAYS "NO," ASK GRAMMA.

THIS LITTLE BANK IS FOR GOLD IN MY PURSE WHEN THERE'S SILVER IN MY HAIR.

CANDY CLOWN

Level of difficulty: * * * * *

MATERIALS: Cardboard, fabric scraps, 2½ inch plastic flower pots, empty baby food jars, empty medicine cups, ball trim or cotton balls, ric rac (optional), colored paper (red, pink, blue, purple, yellow), craft glue, brush, scissors, pinking shears, candy and gum.

APPLICATIONS: Candy clowns are sure to bring smiles to children's faces. Seniors can give them to their grandchildren, and children can give them to their friends. The clowns are made from items usually thrown away. The baby food jars are easily found in hospital or nursing home kitchens. Patients especially like to save their medicine cups for craft projects. And nurseries are always glad to give away their used plastic pots. Just ask for them.

PREPARATION BEFORE CRAFT SESSION: Using the cardboard, cut one hat base and one foot base for each clown. Then with the pinking shears and fabric, cut five collars, one hat, one hat base, and one foot base for each clown. Cut out eyes, hair, cheeks, and lips from the colored paper.

CRAFT SESSION: Glue the fabric to the cardboard foot base and hat base. Trim the feet with ric rac and ball trim or cotton balls. Glue the five cloth collars to the outside lip of the jar. Glue the jar onto the foot base. Fill the jar with candy and gum. Turn the flower pot upside down and glue on the face and hair. Glue the fabric hat around the medicine cup, which has also been turned upside down. Then glue the hat to the hat base and then the completed hat to the bottom of the flower pot. Attach a ball trim or cotton ball to the tip of the hat, and put the clown face *lid* on the candy-filled jar.

CANDY CLOWN

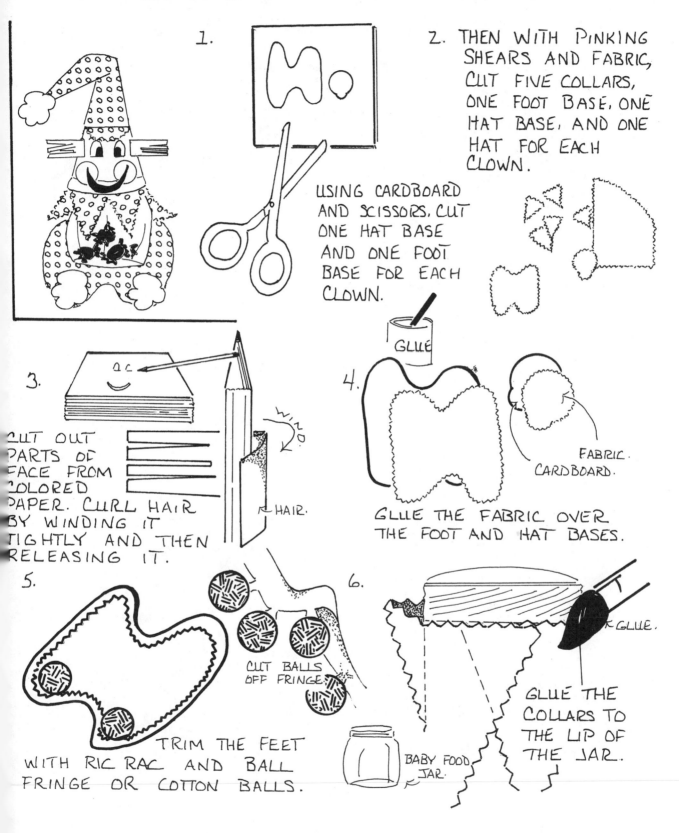

1.

2. THEN WITH PINKING SHEARS AND FABRIC, CUT FIVE COLLARS, ONE FOOT BASE, ONE HAT BASE, AND ONE HAT FOR EACH CLOWN.

USING CARDBOARD AND SCISSORS, CUT ONE HAT BASE AND ONE FOOT BASE FOR EACH CLOWN.

GLUE

3.

CUT OUT PARTS OF FACE FROM COLORED PAPER. CURL HAIR BY WINDING IT TIGHTLY AND THEN RELEASING IT.

WIND

HAIR.

4.

FABRIC.
CARDBOARD.

GLUE THE FABRIC OVER THE FOOT AND HAT BASES.

5.

CUT BALLS OFF FRINGE.

TRIM THE FEET WITH RIC RAC AND BALL FRINGE OR COTTON BALLS.

6.

GLUE.

GLUE THE COLLARS TO THE LIP OF THE JAR.

BABY FOOD JAR.

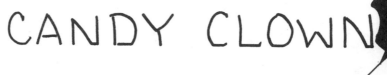

7.

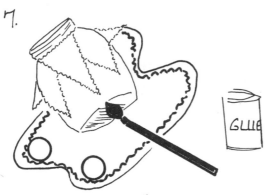

GLUE THE JAR
ONTO THE FOOT BASE.

8.

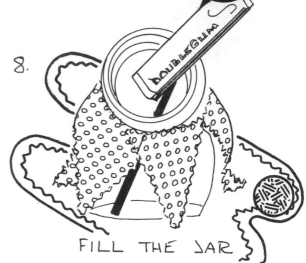

FILL THE JAR
WITH CANDY AND GUM.

9.

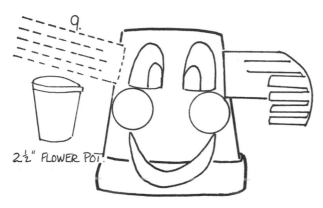

2½" FLOWER POT.

TURN FLOWER POT UPSIDE
DOWN AND GLUE ON FACE.

10.

CONE. →

WRAP FABRIC
HAT AROUND
UPSIDE DOWN
MEDICINE CUP
AND GLUE IT
TO FORM A
CONE.

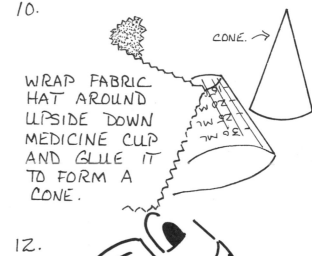

11.

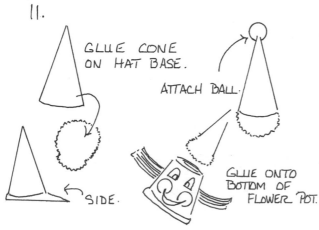

GLUE CONE
ON HAT BASE.

ATTACH BALL.

GLUE ONTO
BOTTOM OF
FLOWER POT.

← SIDE.

FINISH THE HAT.

12.

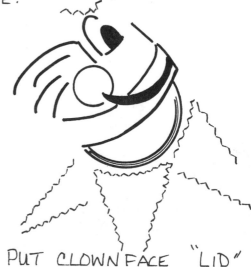

PUT CLOWN FACE "LID"
ON CANDY FILLED JAR.

PATTERNS FOR CANDY CLOWN

HAT BASE.

FOOT BASE.

HAT.

COLLAR.

EYES.

HAIR.
(CUT AND CURL.)

CHEEKS.

MOUTH.

BUTTON-ON DOGGIES

Level of difficulty: ***—****

MATERIALS: Scissors, buttons, needles, thread, single-edged razors, thimble, leatherette samples or heavy oil cloth, adhesive tape, felt marking pen.

APPLICATIONS: These cute *button-on doggies* are used to lengthen shoulder straps on overalls and suspenders. They are useful gifts for young mamas who do not have time to re-sew buttons.

PREPARATION BEFORE CRAFT SESSION: Draw sets of doggies on the leatherette and cut them out. Place adhesive tape on the backs of the doggies as illustrated. Using a razor blade, *slice* a button hole in the head of each doggie. Mark the location for each button.

CRAFT SESSION: Sew buttons on the bottom of each doggie. Make lots of sets.

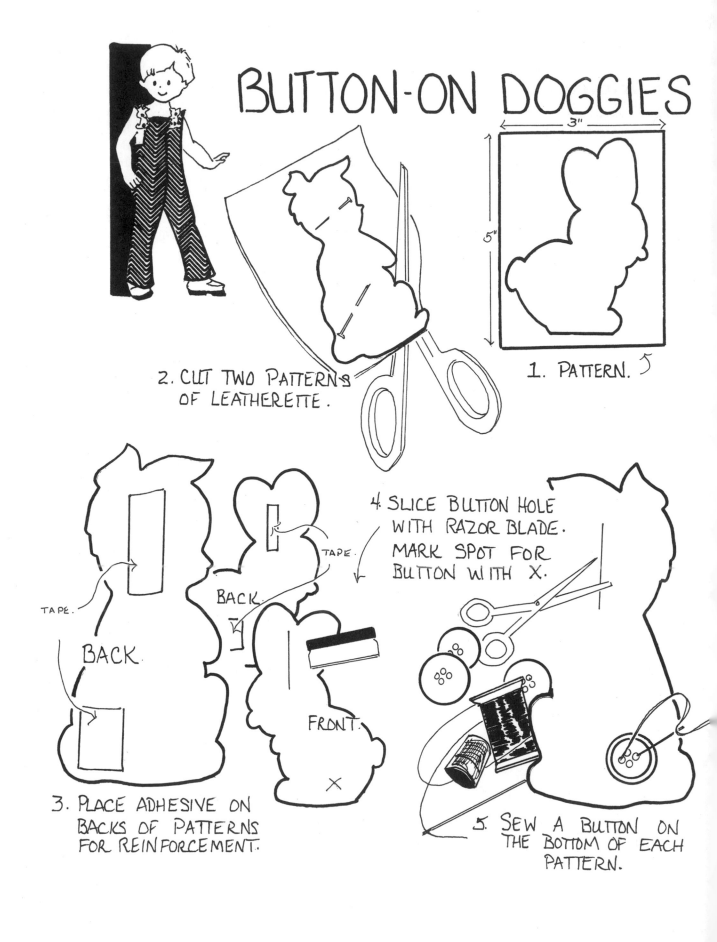

BUTTON-ON DOGGIES

1. PATTERN.

2. CUT TWO PATTERNS OF LEATHERETTE.

3. PLACE ADHESIVE ON BACKS OF PATTERNS FOR REINFORCEMENT.

BACK.

TAPE.

BACK.

TAPE.

4. SLICE BUTTON HOLE WITH RAZOR BLADE. MARK SPOT FOR BUTTON WITH X.

FRONT.

5. SEW A BUTTON ON THE BOTTOM OF EACH PATTERN.

3"

5"

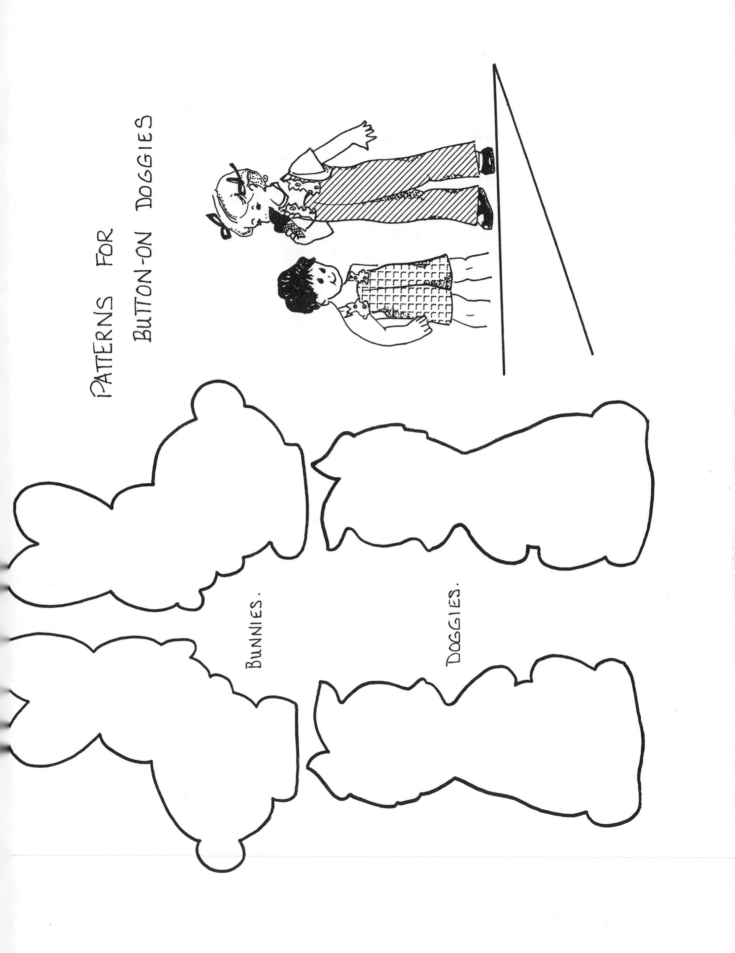

PATTERNS FOR BUTTON-ON DOGGIES

BUNNIES.

DOGGIES.

SHOE TREES

Level of difficulty: *—*****

MATERIALS: Pinking shears, ribbon, old stockings, fabric scraps, string or heavy thread, small decorative ornaments (optional).

APPLICATIONS: Every family member will appreciate shoe trees. Make satin ones for ladies and corduroy ones for men, or use pastels and plaids. Tie bows around the ladies'; tie knots around the men's.

PREPARATION BEFORE CRAFT SESSION: Cut two matching circles of fabric 14 inches in diameter with a pinking shears for each pair of shoe trees.

CRAFT SESSION: Stuff the toes of the old stockings with fabric scraps and tie with thread. Cover the stuffed stockings with the circles of cloth. Gather the edges together and tie them with ribbon. Pull the edges so that the fabric becomes taut over the stocking. Insert ornaments under the ribbon if desired.

SHOE TREES

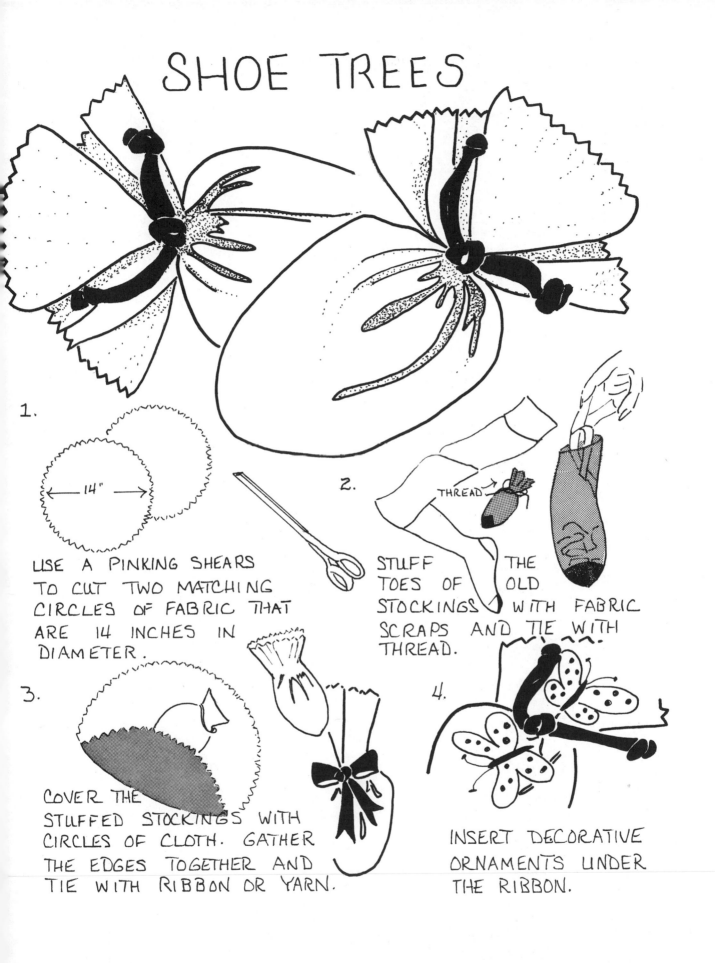

1. USE A PINKING SHEARS TO CUT TWO MATCHING CIRCLES OF FABRIC THAT ARE 14 INCHES IN DIAMETER.

2. STUFF THE TOES OF OLD STOCKINGS WITH FABRIC SCRAPS AND TIE WITH THREAD.

THREAD

3. COVER THE STUFFED STOCKINGS WITH CIRCLES OF CLOTH. GATHER THE EDGES TOGETHER AND TIE WITH RIBBON OR YARN.

4. INSERT DECORATIVE ORNAMENTS UNDER THE RIBBON.

CHAPTER SIX

Craft Projects for Use by Agencies

TOY ANIMALS AND TOY BUILDINGS

Level of difficulty: ***—*****

MATERIALS: Wood scraps, 00 sandpaper, craft glue, water base paint in a variety of colors, brushes, felt marking pens.

APPLICATIONS: These imaginative toys are appreciated during the holiday season by volunteer agencies and by community clubs that sponsor programs for the needy. You can also donate the toys to the Salvation Army or to church nurseries. This is a great project for men, women, and children alike.

PREPARATION BEFORE CRAFT SESSION: You may want to glue together some animals or buildings for those people who do not want to wait for glue to dry before painting. See craft session for instructions.

CRAFT SESSION: Pick out some interesting pieces of wood that look somewhat like animal shapes or parts of buildings. Fit the pieces together to create imaginary animals or buildings. After you have selected the pieces of wood, sand them all smooth with 00 sandpaper. Then fit the parts together again, and glue them in place. Paint them any colors you wish. Allow this first coat of paint to dry. Then use paint or felt pens to draw detail designs with other colors. Do this very free hand. Make lots of toys.

TOY ANIMALS

WOOD SCRAPS FROM LUMBER YARD.

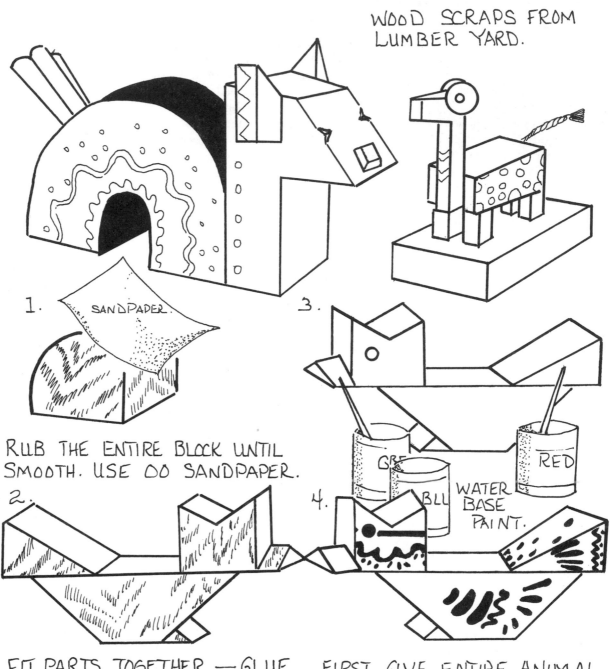

1. SANDPAPER

RUB THE ENTIRE BLOCK UNTIL SMOOTH. USE OO SANDPAPER.

2. FIT PARTS TOGETHER — GLUE OR NAIL IN PLACE.

3.

4. WATER BASE PAINT.

GRE BLU RED

FIRST GIVE ENTIRE ANIMAL A COAT OF PAINT. DRY. THEN PAINT DETAIL DESIGN.

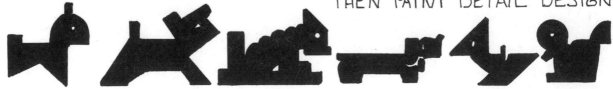

TOY BUILDINGS

USE WOOD SCRAPS
FOR THESE CREATIVE
TOYS AND MODELS.

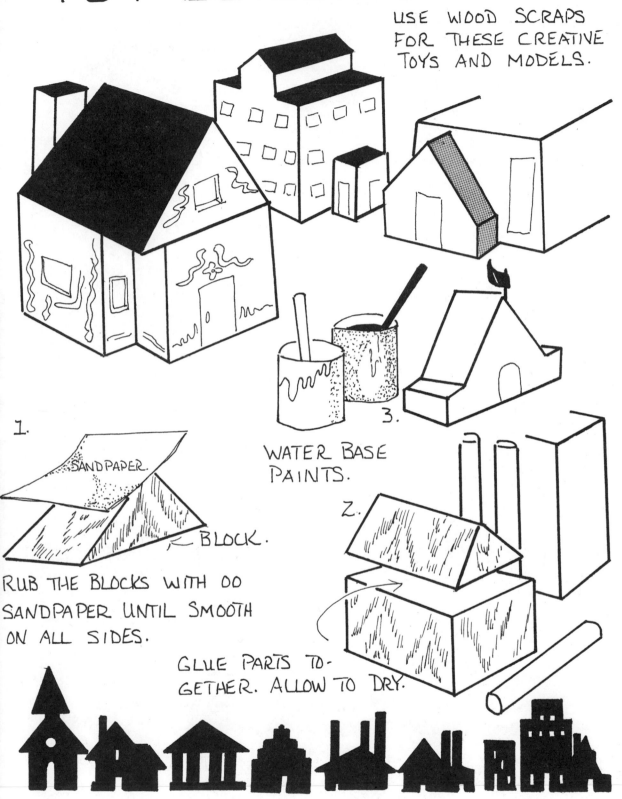

WATER BASE
PAINTS.

1.

SANDPAPER.

BLOCK.

RUB THE BLOCKS WITH OO
SANDPAPER UNTIL SMOOTH
ON ALL SIDES.

2.

3.

GLUE PARTS TO-
GETHER. ALLOW TO DRY.

TREE TRIMMING

Level of difficulty: *—*****

MATERIALS: Colored or white art paper of a medium or heavy weight, scissors, string, narrow ribbon, craft glue, brushes, crayons, felt marking pens in a variety of colors, glue stick, paper punch (metallic paper, gold and silver stars, lace—all optional).

APPLICATIONS: These holiday ornaments may be donated by the dozens to other nursing homes or to your local volunteer bureau.

PREPARATION BEFORE CRAFT SESSION: Cut out dozens of patterns. Distribute one of each design in front of each person and secure them to the table with glue stick.

CRAFT SESSION: Decorate the patterns with crayon or felt markers. Sign each pattern when complete. Follow the directions on the charts for folding and gluing. Add gold and silver stars, lace, and ribbons if you wish, or make the stars of metallic paper.

TREE TRIMMING BIRDS

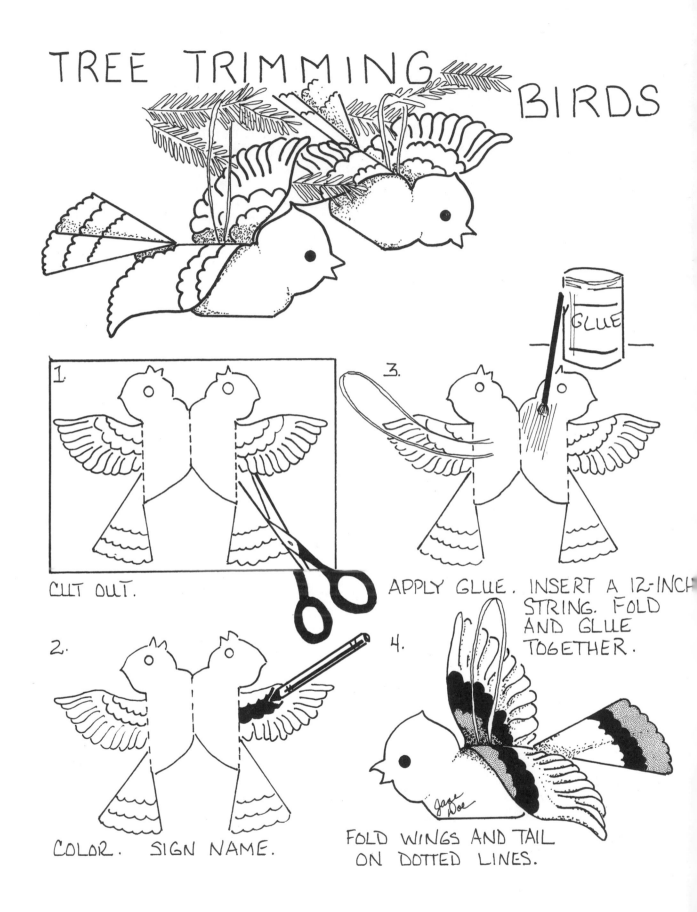

1. CUT OUT.

2. COLOR. SIGN NAME.

3. APPLY GLUE. INSERT A 12-INCH STRING. FOLD AND GLUE TOGETHER.

4. FOLD WINGS AND TAIL ON DOTTED LINES.

GLUE

PATTERN FOR TREE TRIMMING.
BIRDS

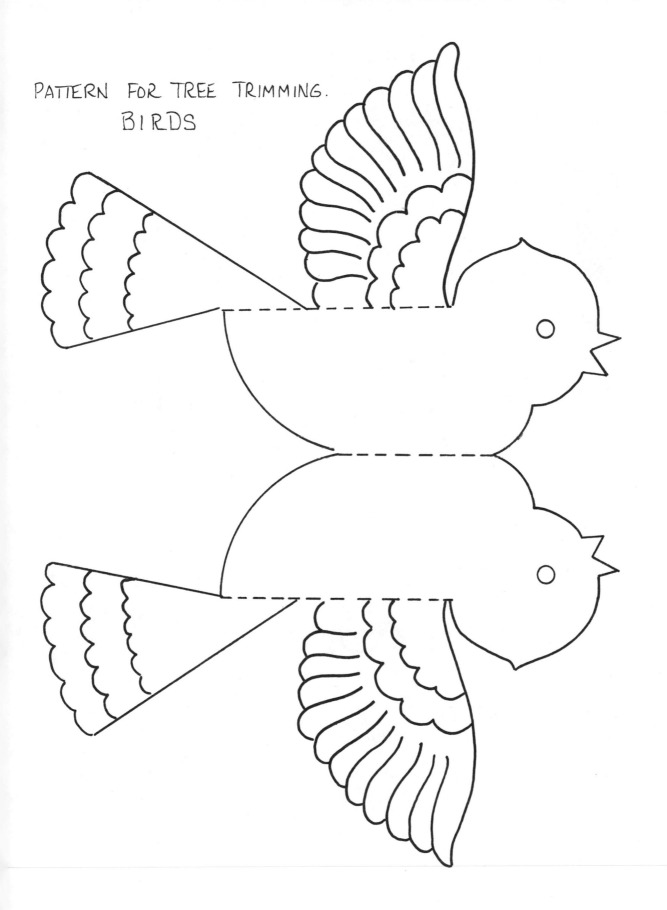

TREE ANGEL

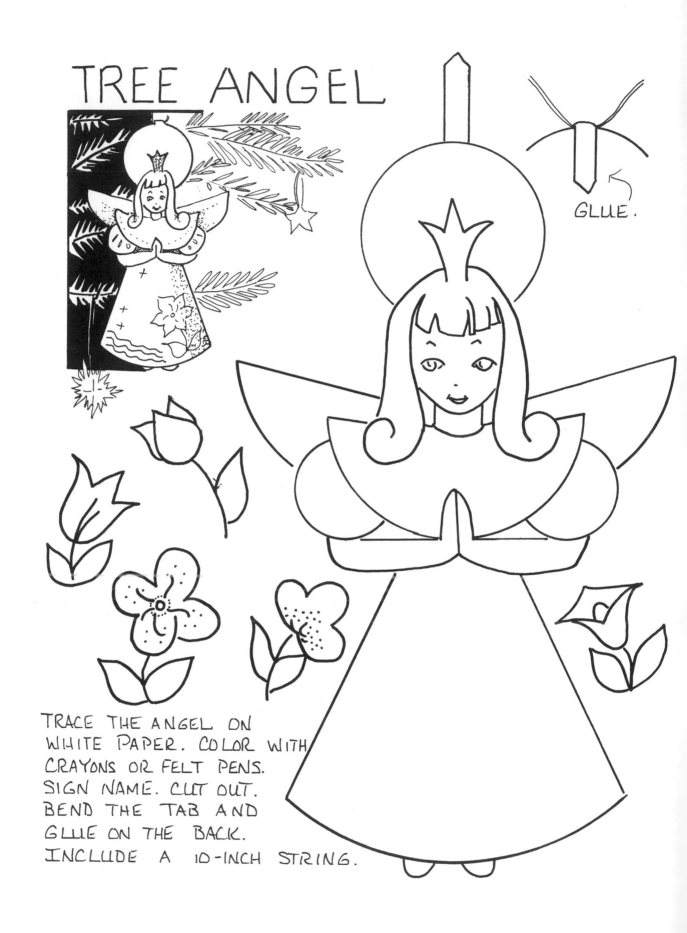

GLUE.

TRACE THE ANGEL ON
WHITE PAPER. COLOR WITH
CRAYONS OR FELT PENS.
SIGN NAME. CUT OUT.
BEND THE TAB AND
GLUE ON THE BACK.
INCLUDE A 10-INCH STRING.

TREE ANGEL

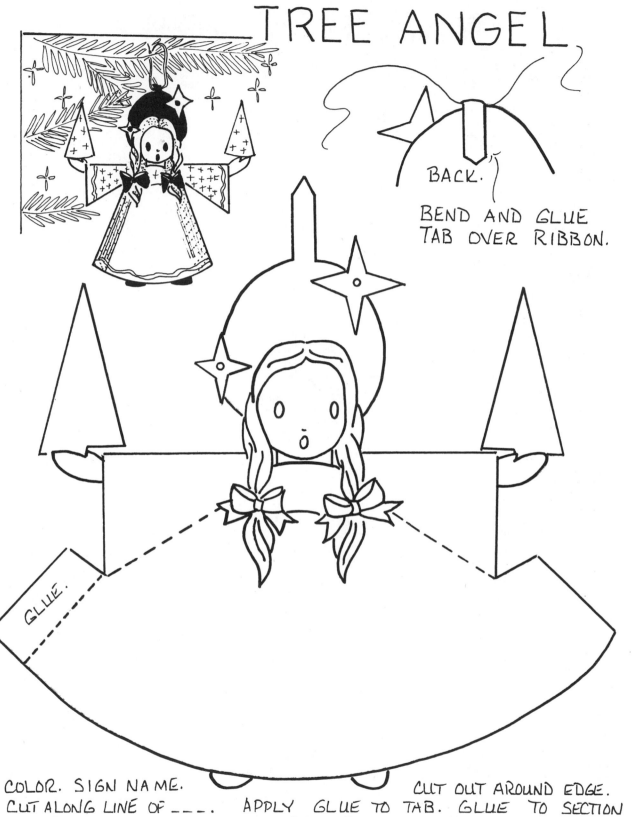

BACK.

BEND AND GLUE
TAB OVER RIBBON.

GLUE.

COLOR. SIGN NAME.
CUT ALONG LINE OF _ _ _ _.   APPLY   GLUE TO TAB. GLUE   TO SECTION
ON OPPOSITE   SIDE   TO   FORM "CONE" FOR SKIRT.

CUT OUT AROUND EDGE.

PAPER STARS

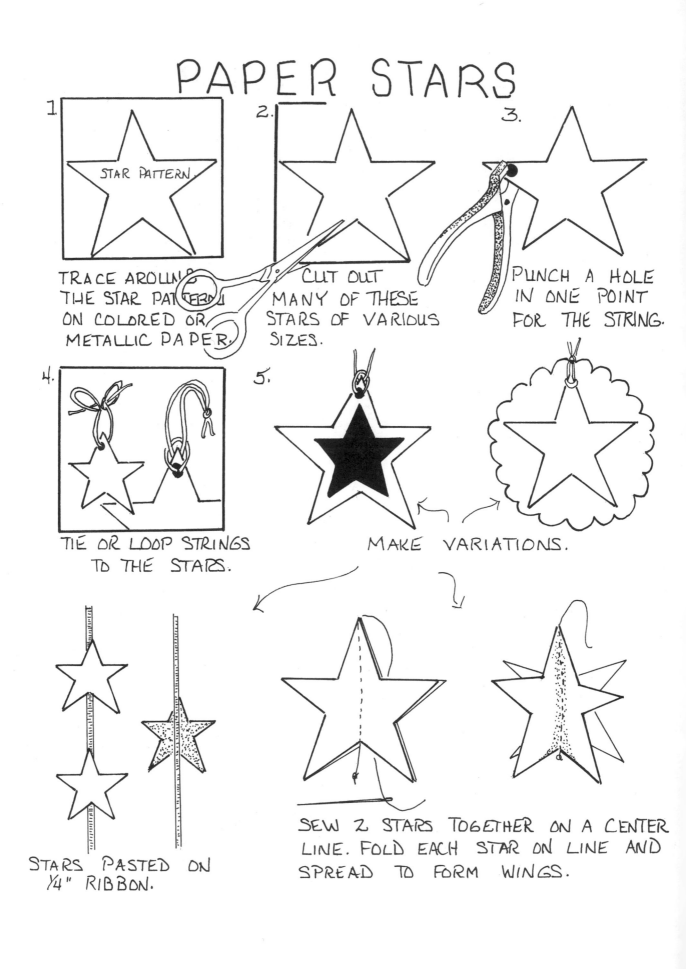

1. STAR PATTERN. — TRACE AROUND THE STAR PATTERN ON COLORED OR METALLIC PAPER.

2. CUT OUT MANY OF THESE STARS OF VARIOUS SIZES.

3. PUNCH A HOLE IN ONE POINT FOR THE STRING.

4. TIE OR LOOP STRINGS TO THE STARS.

5. MAKE VARIATIONS.

STARS PASTED ON ¼" RIBBON.

SEW 2 STARS TOGETHER ON A CENTER LINE. FOLD EACH STAR ON LINE AND SPREAD TO FORM WINGS.

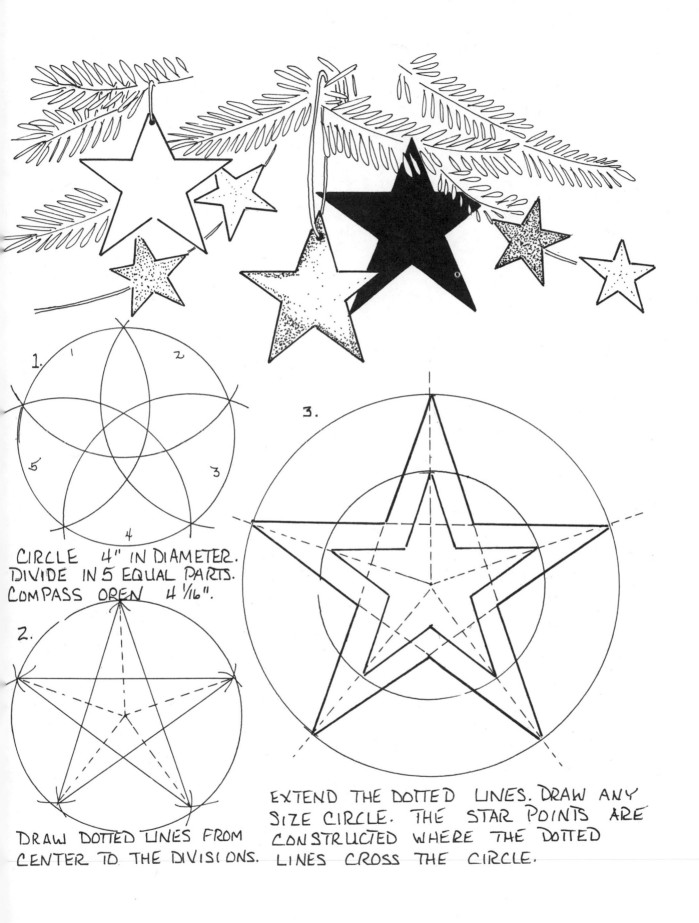

1.

CIRCLE 4" IN DIAMETER.
DIVIDE IN 5 EQUAL PARTS.
COMPASS OPEN 4 1/16".

2.

3.

DRAW DOTTED LINES FROM
CENTER TO THE DIVISIONS.

EXTEND THE DOTTED LINES. DRAW ANY
SIZE CIRCLE. THE STAR POINTS ARE
CONSTRUCTED WHERE THE DOTTED
LINES CROSS THE CIRCLE.

ORNAMENTS

Level of difficulty: *****

MATERIALS: Glitter, craft glue, empty margarine tubs, large sequins, straight pins, 6-inch Styrofoam ball, metallic ribbon or cord, empty medicine cups, scissors, wet paper towels or a wet washcloth.

APPLICATIONS: These ornaments are spectacular. Donate them to your local fire department and police station at holiday time to express appreciation for the expertise they demonstrate all year in help for the disabled and handicapped.

PREPARATION BEFORE CRAFT SESSION: Cut a piece of ribbon 24 inches long. Fold the ribbon in half to make a long loop, and secure it to the Styrofoam ball with glue. Sprinkle glitter over the excess glue for decoration. Pour glue into one margarine tub and glitter into another. Stick straight pins through the large sequins and put them in a margarine tub.

CRAFT SESSION: Dip the rim of a medicine cup lightly in glue. Then dip it in glitter. Now dip the bottom of the same cup in glue and secure it on the Styrofoam ball with a straight pin and sequin. Repeat this process until the entire ball is covered with medicine cups, which have been placed as close to each other as possible. Use the wet towels or wash cloth whenever fingers get sticky.

ORNAMENTS

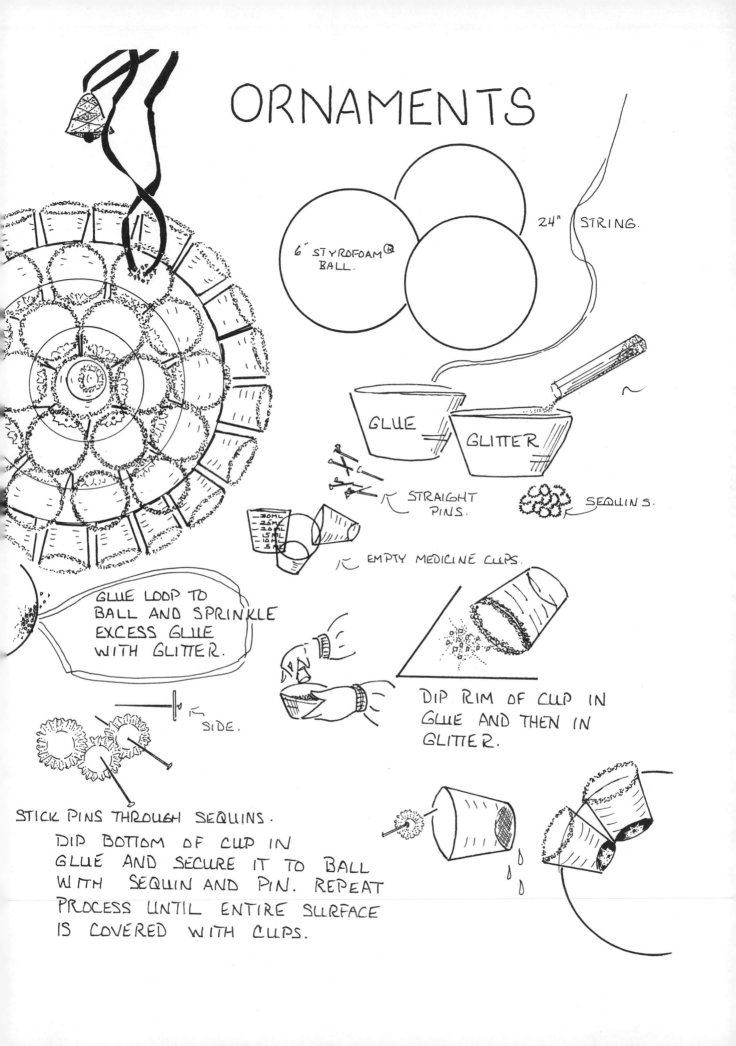

6" STYROFOAM® BALL.

24" STRING.

GLUE

GLITTER

STRAIGHT PINS.

SEQUINS.

EMPTY MEDICINE CUPS.

GLUE LOOP TO BALL AND SPRINKLE EXCESS GLUE WITH GLITTER.

SIDE.

DIP RIM OF CUP IN GLUE AND THEN IN GLITTER.

STICK PINS THROUGH SEQUINS.
DIP BOTTOM OF CUP IN GLUE AND SECURE IT TO BALL WITH SEQUIN AND PIN. REPEAT PROCESS UNTIL ENTIRE SURFACE IS COVERED WITH CUPS.

HOLIDAY CARDS

Level of difficulty: *—**

MATERIALS: Colored construction paper, felt marking pens, ribbon, glue stick, paper punch, scissors (holiday stickers, optional).

APPLICATIONS: These simple cards are appreciated by your governmental volunteer agency, which will distribute the cards on meal trays to other hospitals and nursing homes.

PREPARATION BEFORE CRAFT SESSION: Cut ribbon into 12-inch lengths. Trace the outline of the pattern of the cards on a folded piece of construction paper. Cut it out double, but do not cut along the folded edge. Make an eyelet hole in the position indicated. Using glue stick, secure a card in front of each person.

CRAFT SESSION: Decorate the cards with felt pens. Some people may prefer to put holiday stickers on the cards rather than draw. Write greetings inside each card, and have each person sign his name. Tie the card with a 12-inch length of narrow ribbon.

HOLIDAY CARDS

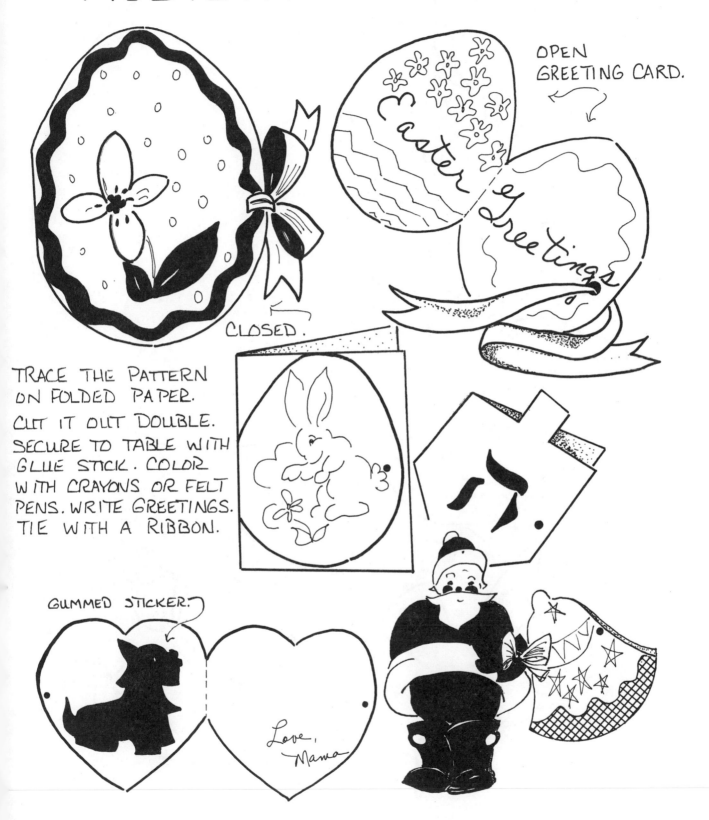

OPEN GREETING CARD.

CLOSED.

Easter greetings

TRACE THE PATTERN ON FOLDED PAPER. CUT IT OUT DOUBLE. SECURE TO TABLE WITH GLUE STICK. COLOR WITH CRAYONS OR FELT PENS. WRITE GREETINGS. TIE WITH A RIBBON.

GUMMED STICKER.

Love, Mama

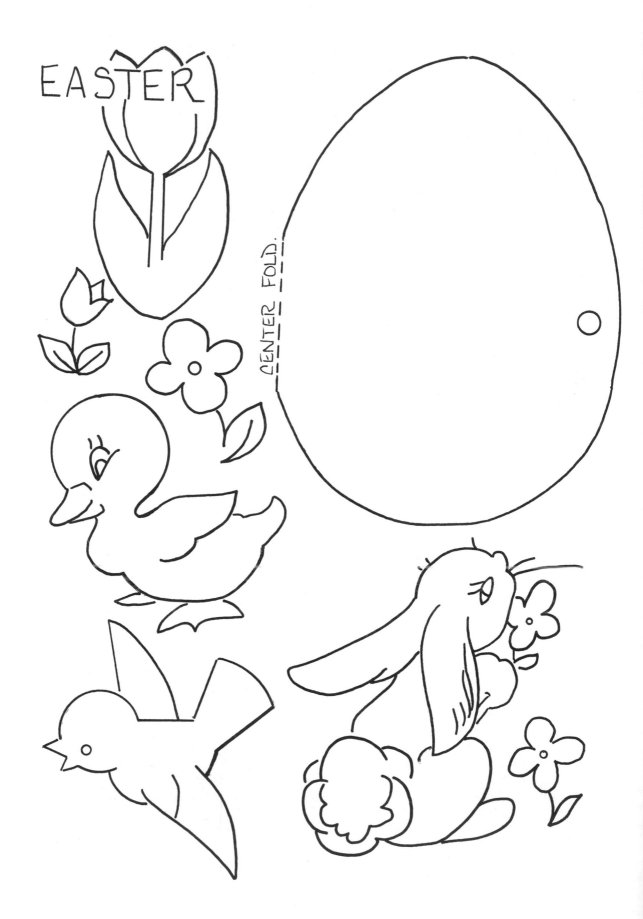

PASSOVER

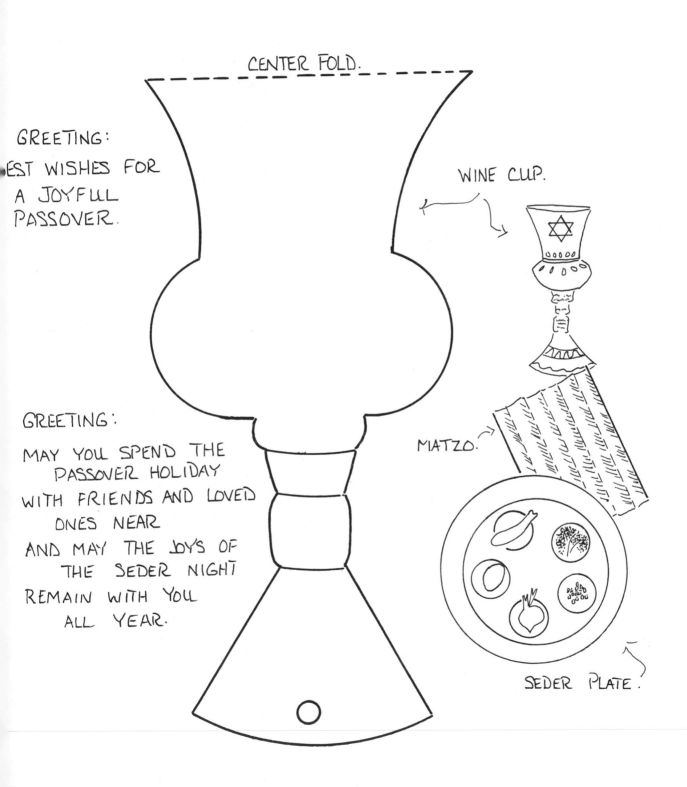

CENTER FOLD.

GREETING:

~EST WISHES FOR
A JOYFUL
PASSOVER.

GREETING:

MAY YOU SPEND THE
   PASSOVER HOLIDAY
WITH FRIENDS AND LOVED
   ONES NEAR
AND MAY THE JOYS OF
   THE SEDER NIGHT
REMAIN WITH YOU
   ALL YEAR.

WINE CUP.

MATZO.

SEDER PLATE.

VALENTINES DAY

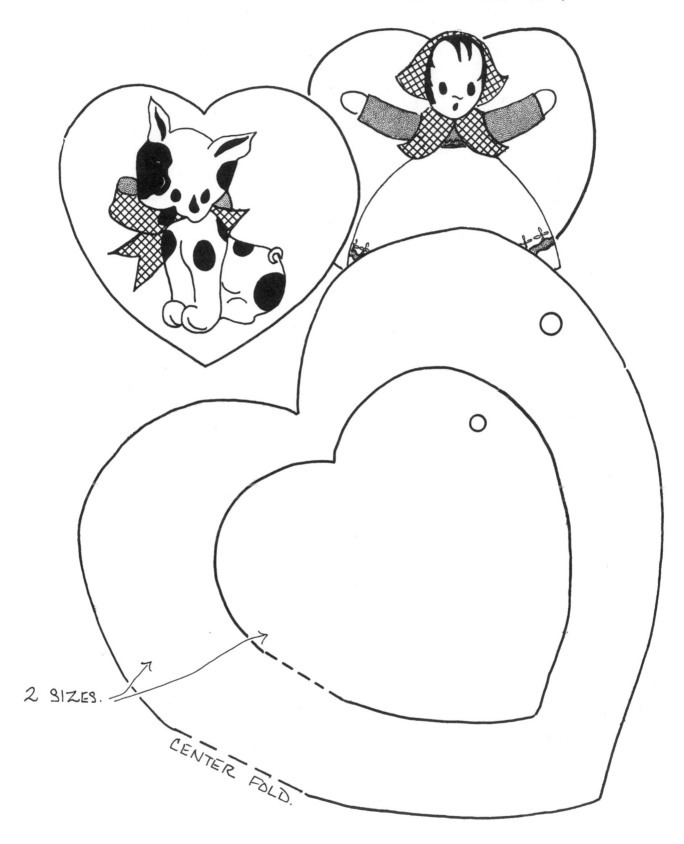

2 SIZES.

CENTER FOLD.

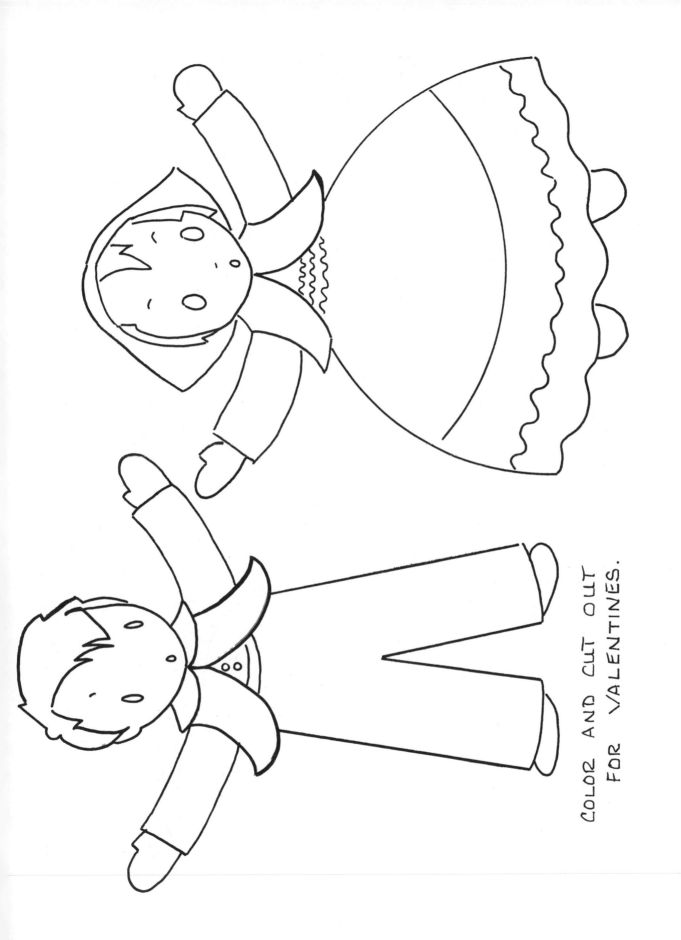

COLOR AND CUT OUT
FOR VALENTINES.

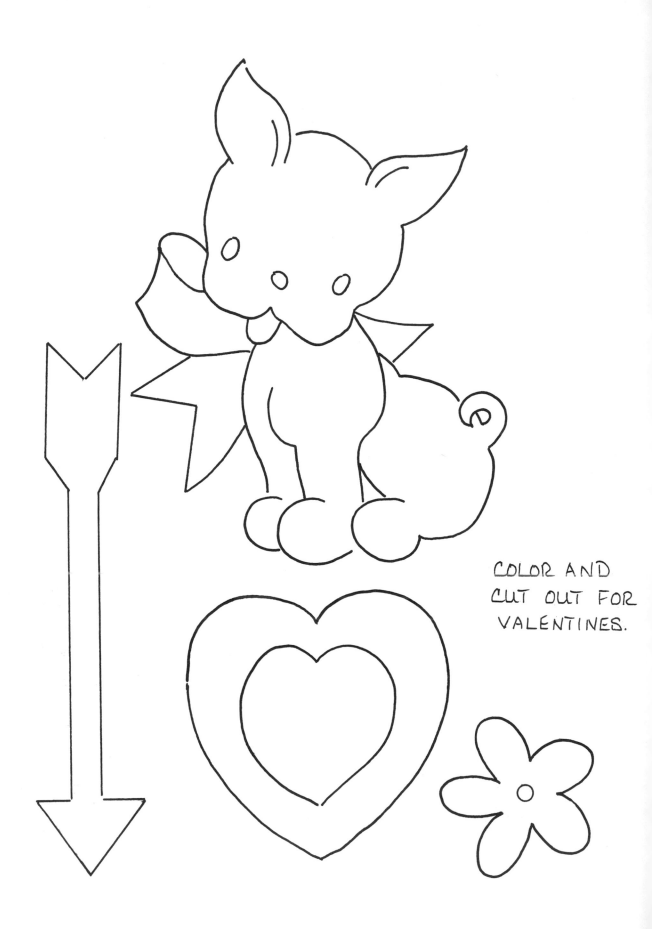

COLOR AND
CUT OUT FOR
VALENTINES.

CHRISTMAS

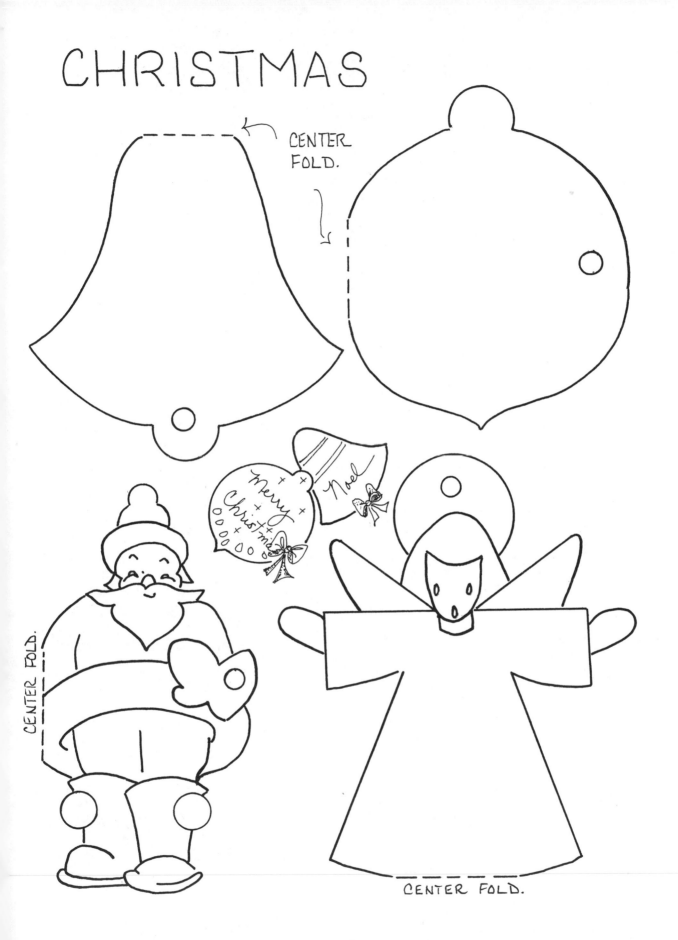

CENTER FOLD.

CENTER FOLD.

CENTER FOLD.

CHRISTMAS

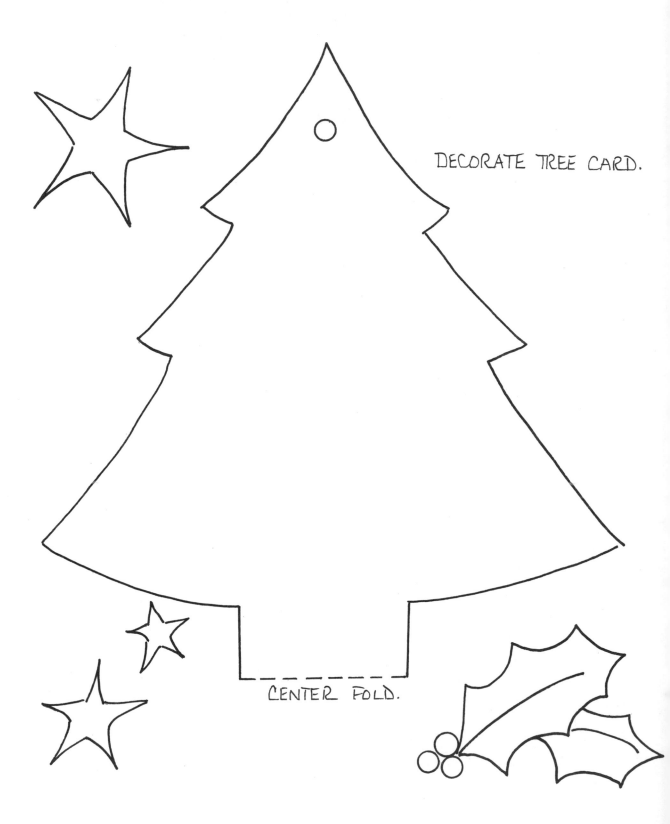

DECORATE TREE CARD.

CENTER FOLD.

CHANUKAH

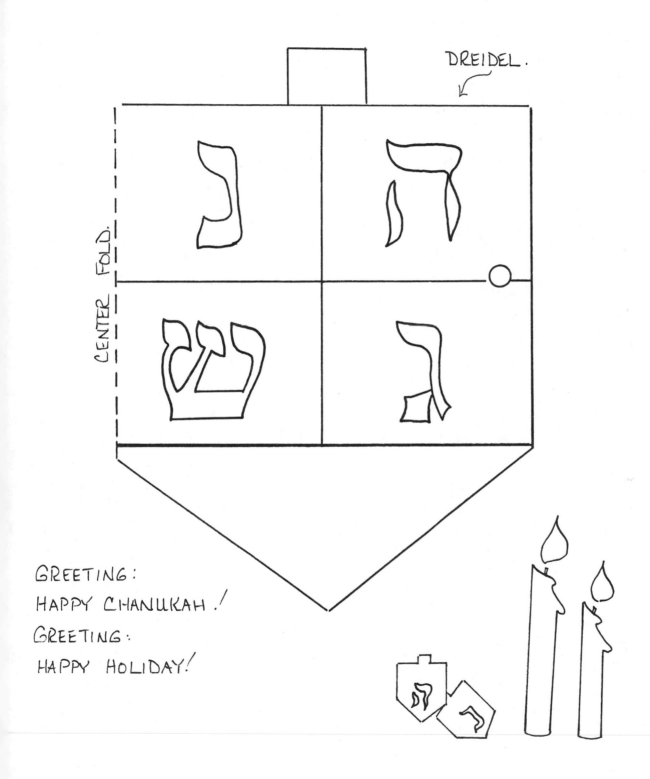

DREIDEL.

CENTER FOLD.

GREETING:
HAPPY CHANUKAH.!
GREETING:
HAPPY HOLIDAY!

JEWISH NEW YEAR

GREETING:
   L'SHANA TOVA
   HAPPY NEW YEAR

GREETING:

ON ROSH HASHONA
   EVERY YEAR,
WE HEAR THE SHOFAR
   LOUD AND CLEAR.
ON YOM KIPPUR WE
   HEAR IT TOO,
"A HAPPY YEAR!" IT
   CALLS TO YOU.

CENTER FOLD.

SHOFAR.

OPEN.

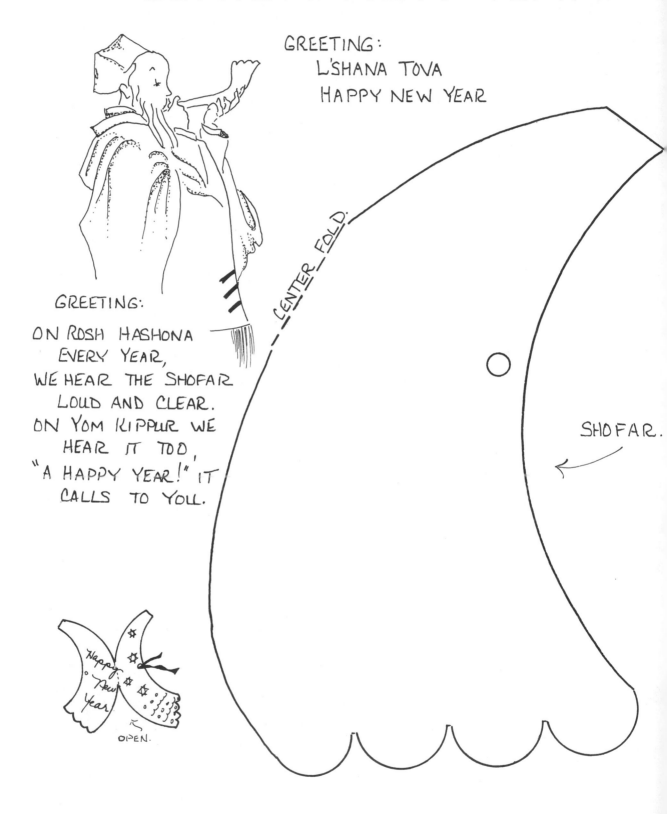

SCISSORS CANS

Level of difficulty: *—***

MATERIALS: Fabric scraps, pinking shears, craft glue, brushes, empty 16 ounce frozen concentrated juice cans (makes ½ gallon), ric rac or ball fringe.

APPLICATIONS: Any government agency can use lots of scissors cans for secretaries' desks. The nice tall height of this size juice can makes a very stable container which holds lots of scissors and will not tip over. (I carry one around in my craft supply box so I do not have to dig to find my shears.) You might want to donate pretty cans to fabric stores which would in turn supply you with samples or remnants.

PREPARATION BEFORE CRAFT SESSION: Using a pinking shears, cut fabric into pieces 6¼ inches by 9 inches.

CRAFT SESSION: Brush glue on the can. Wrap fabric around the can. Decorate the top with ric rac or ball fringe.

SCISSORS CAN

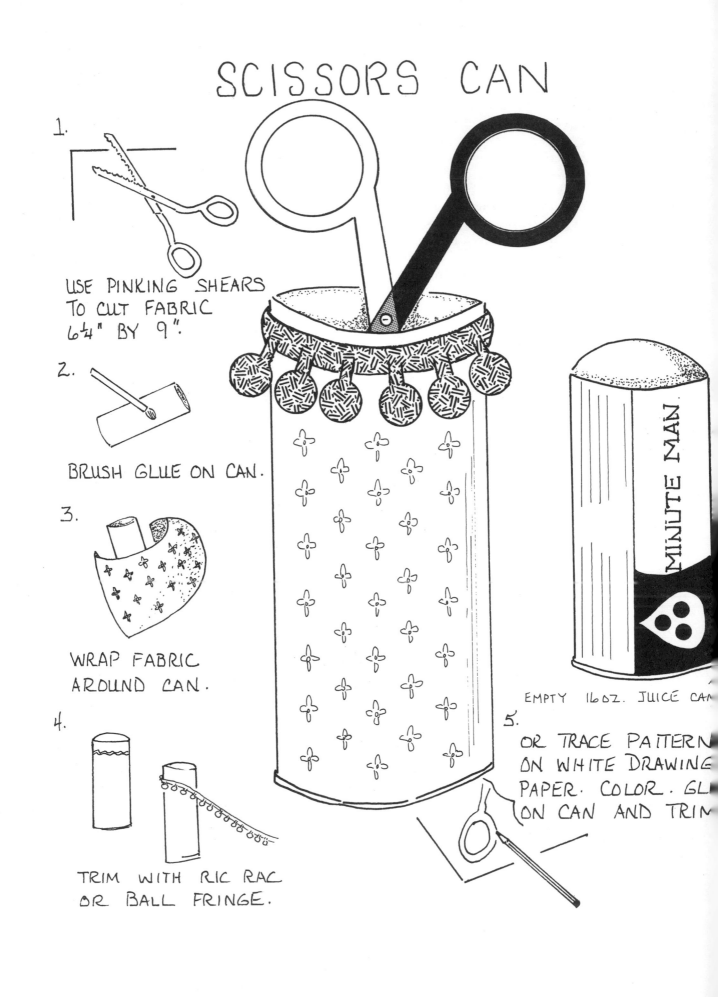

1. USE PINKING SHEARS TO CUT FABRIC 6¼" BY 9".

2. BRUSH GLUE ON CAN.

3. WRAP FABRIC AROUND CAN.

4. TRIM WITH RIC RAC OR BALL FRINGE.

EMPTY 16 OZ. JUICE CAN

MINUTE MAN

5. OR TRACE PATTERN ON WHITE DRAWING PAPER. COLOR. GL ON CAN AND TRIM

TRIM. →

PATTERN FOR PAPER - COVERED SCISSORS CAN.

JINGLES AND JANGLES

Level of difficulty: ***—*****

MATERIALS: Package handles, fine wire, hammer, small pieces of plywood (optional), bottle caps, nails, rattles, or bells.

APPLICATIONS: These musical jingles and jangles are enjoyable both to make and use. They are grand for nursing home rhythm bands, family service agencies or orphanages, and government daycare and preschool programs. Men especially will like to do the hammer and nail work in making these.

PREPARATION BEFORE CRAFT SESSION: For each package handle, flatten six or eight bottle caps by tapping the edges down toward the outside with a hammer. Cut the wire into 6-inch lengths. Leave some bottle caps unprepared for those people who are able to flatten them.

CRAFT SESSION: Pry loose the cork that is in the center of each bottle cap. If you are not working on a work table or bench, place the caps on plywood. Then with a hammer and nail, punch a hole in the center of each bottle cap. Fasten one end of the wire to one side of the package handle, string the bottle caps on the wire, and fasten the other end of the wire to the opposite side of the package handle. Shake the handle for jingles and jangles. Try various metallic objects like nails, bells, screws, and rattles instead of bottle caps.

JINGLES AND JANGLES

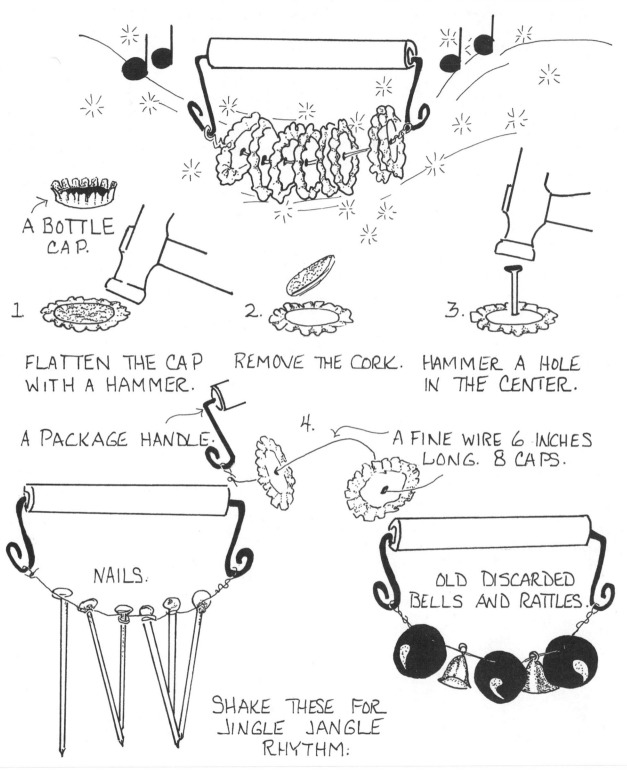

A BOTTLE CAP.

1. FLATTEN THE CAP WITH A HAMMER.

2. REMOVE THE CORK.

3. HAMMER A HOLE IN THE CENTER.

A PACKAGE HANDLE.

4. A FINE WIRE 6 INCHES LONG. 8 CAPS.

NAILS.

OLD DISCARDED BELLS AND RATTLES.

SHAKE THESE FOR JINGLE JANGLE RHYTHM.

BOOKMARKS

Level of difficulty: ***—*****

MATERIALS: Colored art paper, clear contact paper, scissors, pinking shears, paper punch, narrow satin ribbon (or bias binding, ric rac, etc.), dried flowers and leaves, straight pin, black felt marking pen.

APPLICATIONS: The illustration shows how to make bookmarks by using materials from nature. After trying these, you can make interesting notepaper, pictures, etc. Donate the bookmarks to the public library or a nearby school.

PREPARATION BEFORE CRAFT SESSION: Cut 2 x 6 inch strips of colored art paper. For each strip of paper, cut two pieces of contact paper the same size. Also cut 12-inch strips of narrow ribbon. Have a nice collection of dried blossoms, leaves, weeds, or ferns. To dry plants, place the picked leaves or blossoms (preferably flat ones) in an old phone book or paperback or between sheets of newspaper. Let them stay untouched for one week. They will then be ready for use. Generally, have twice as much as is needed, because feeble hands often break the delicate dried leaves and blossoms. Clover and ferns are especially nice.

CRAFT SESSION: Have each person choose the color of paper he desires and the dried flowers and leaves he likes. Then have the individual arrange the flowers in a pleasing design and sign his name. Help him peel the contact paper and press it down on the leaves and paper. Use a pin to puncture the contact paper to get out any air bubbles. Repeat the design process on the other side. Trim all four edges with a pinking shears. Punch a hole at one end with a paper punch. Insert a ribbon by folding it in half and looping it through the hole.

BOOKMARKS

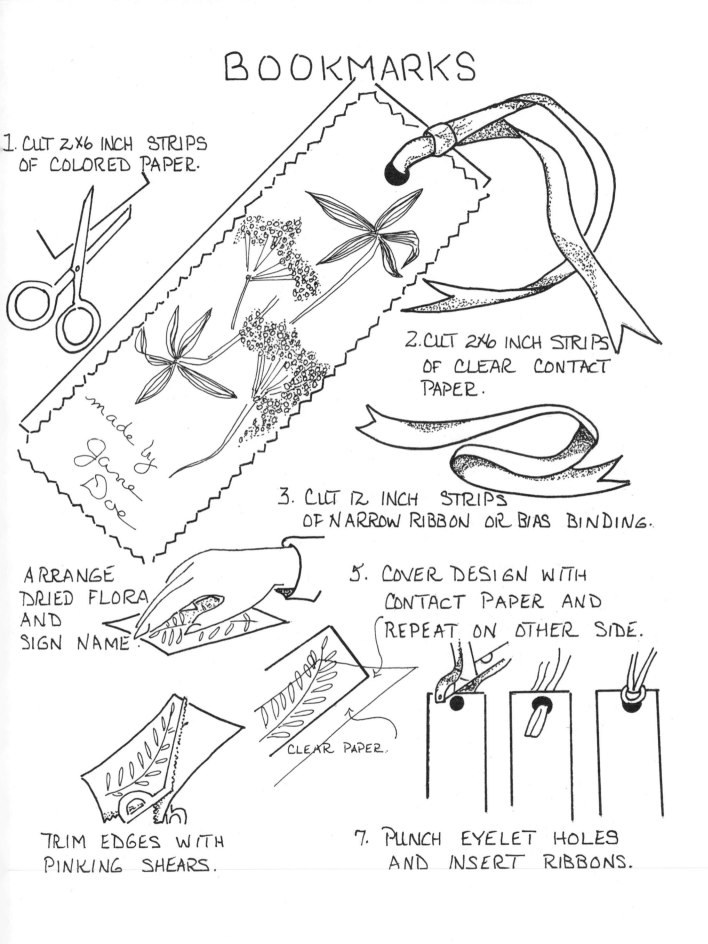

1. CUT 2X6 INCH STRIPS OF COLORED PAPER.

2. CUT 2X6 INCH STRIPS OF CLEAR CONTACT PAPER.

3. CUT 12 INCH STRIPS OF NARROW RIBBON OR BIAS BINDING.

ARRANGE DRIED FLORA AND SIGN NAME.

made by Jane Doe

5. COVER DESIGN WITH CONTACT PAPER AND REPEAT ON OTHER SIDE.

CLEAR PAPER.

TRIM EDGES WITH PINKING SHEARS.

7. PUNCH EYELET HOLES AND INSERT RIBBONS.

NUT BASKETS

Level of difficulty: ***—*****

MATERIALS: Colored construction paper, white drawing paper, crayons, scissors, glue, nuts, glue stick.

APPLICATIONS: Send these little Thanksgiving baskets to a local governmental volunteer agency for distribution to needy families.

PREPARATION BEFORE CRAFT SESSION: Cut the square pattern out of some heavy colored paper. Cut on the heavy line; mark the broken lines and shaded area. Cut out turkeys or apples of white paper. Using glue stick, secure turkeys and apples to the table in front of each person.

CRAFT SESSION: Fold the squares to form a box. Do this by always folding toward the center and slipping the shaded squares to the outside. Apply glue to the shaded areas and form the shape of a box. Crayon the apples and turkeys, and glue them to the sides of the box. Fill the baskets with nuts.

NUT BASKET

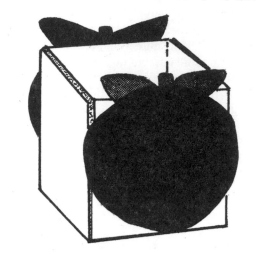

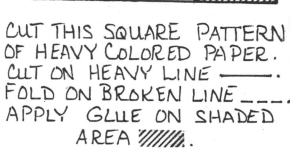

CUT THIS SQUARE PATTERN
OF HEAVY COLORED PAPER.
CUT ON HEAVY LINE ———.
FOLD ON BROKEN LINE ____.
APPLY GLUE ON SHADED
AREA ▨.

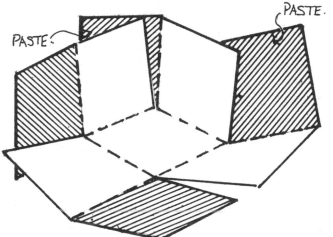

PASTE.   PASTE.

FOLD THE SQUARES TO FORM
A BOX. THE FOLDING IS ALWAYS
TOWARD THE CENTER. THE
GLUED SQUARES SLIP TO THE
OUTSIDE. THEN PRESS FIRMLY.

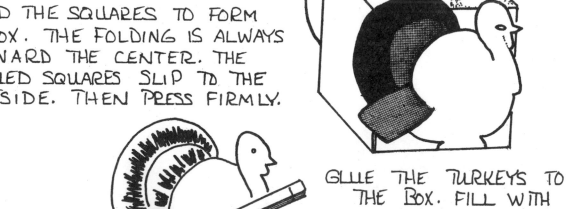

GLUE THE TURKEYS TO
THE BOX. FILL WITH
NUTS.

CUT OUT
AND CRAYON

TURKEYS OR APPLES.

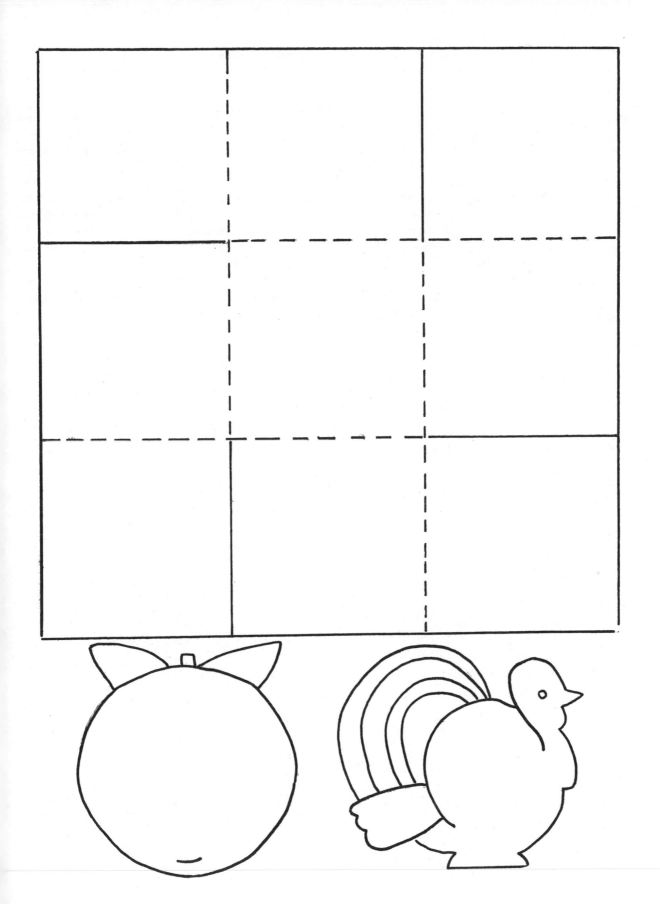

COASTERS

Level of difficulty: *—**

MATERIALS: Sample linoleum or formica tiles (at least 3 inches square), felt, craft glue, art paper, scissors, paper punch, crayons, black felt marking pen, glue stick, brush (magazine pictures, optional).

APPLICATIONS: These colorful coasters are nice for meal trays. You might send some sample coasters to your local radio stations for public service announcements to explain what some disabled people do for others who are also disabled.

PREPARATION BEFORE CRAFT SESSION: Cut art paper into 4½ inch squares. Trace patterns with black felt pens. Using glue stick, secure several squares in front of each person. Also, cut 4 felt corners for each tile.

CRAFT SESSION: Glue a piece of felt on each corner on the backs of the tiles. This gives the coasters a more finished look. Then have each person color his pattern with crayons. Remove the patterns from the table and help cut out the actual picture. Use a paper punch to cut eyes and flower centers. Then glue the pictures to the tiles. Some people prefer to cut out pictures from magazines to glue on the tiles. They are pretty, too.

COASTERS

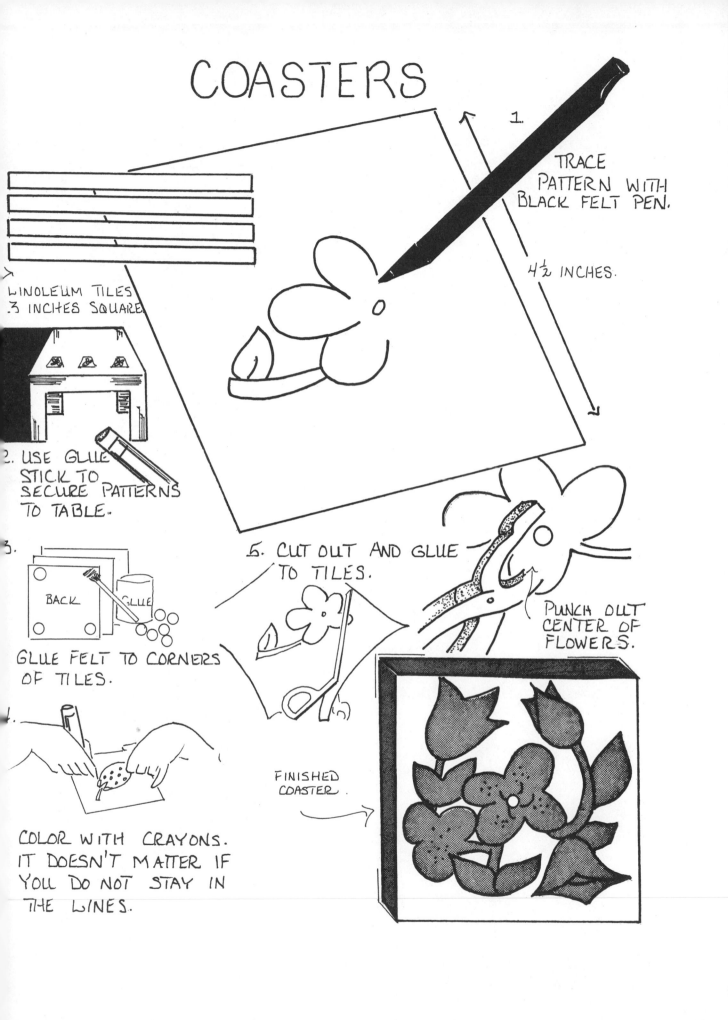

LINOLEUM TILES
.3 INCHES SQUARE.

1. TRACE PATTERN WITH BLACK FELT PEN.

4½ INCHES.

2. USE GLUE STICK TO SECURE PATTERNS TO TABLE.

3. BACK GLUE
GLUE FELT TO CORNERS OF TILES.

5. CUT OUT AND GLUE TO TILES.

PUNCH OUT CENTER OF FLOWERS.

4. COLOR WITH CRAYONS. IT DOESN'T MATTER IF YOU DO NOT STAY IN THE LINES.

FINISHED COASTER.

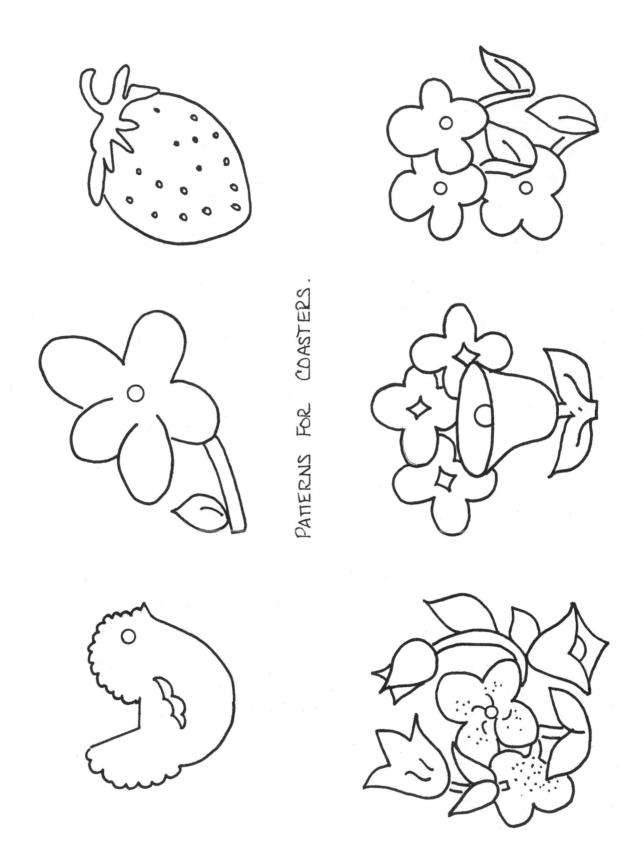

PATTERNS FOR COASTERS.

POTATO PRINT CARDS

Level of difficulty: excellent for *—*****

MATERIALS: Potatoes, knife, red and blue ink pads, white construction paper, ribbon or bias binding (red, white, and blue), felt marking pens (red and blue), paper punch, glue stick.

APPLICATIONS: These simple but eye-catching cards are particularly powerful when sent on the Fourth of July to city, state, and national government representatives to encourage legislation for the disabled and elderly. (Our nursing home had our Congressman present a group of cards to the President welcoming him upon arrival to our city. We received a most grateful letter of appreciation.) The League of Women Voters will provide a list of names, titles, and addresses of all elected officials in government. Most officials personally answer mail, and this is especially exciting to residents of an institution or nursing home.

PREPARATION BEFORE CRAFT SESSION: Cut the potatoes in half. Draw a pattern on each half. Then cut the potato away from the pattern, leaving a relief design on the potato. Fold each piece of paper in half and punch three eyelet holes in each card along the unfolded edge. Cut the ribbon in 12-inch lengths. Using a glue stick, secure a card in front of each person.

CRAFT SESSION: Have each person press the potato on an ink pad and then on this paper. Be careful to keep colors separate. The more frequently the process is repeated, the more attractive is the card. Do not hesitate to overlap pressings of the potato stamp. Then finish decorating the cards with red and blue pens. Write greetings or messages or just sign signatures. Secure the cards with red, white, and blue ribbons looped through the three eyelet holes in each card.

POTATO PRINT CARDS

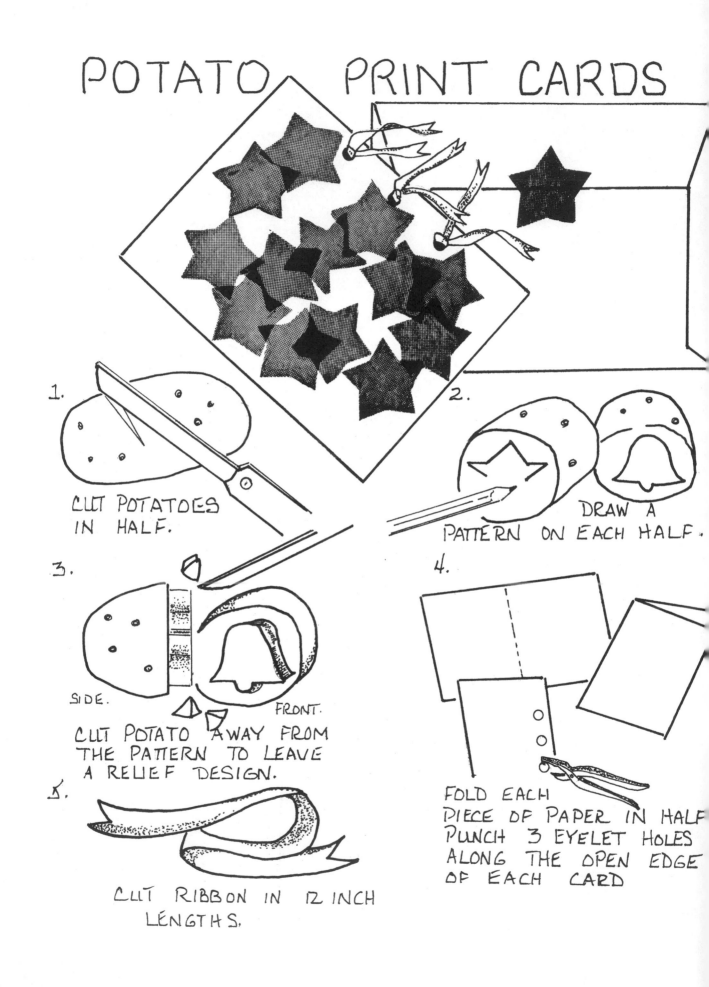

1. CUT POTATOES IN HALF.

2. DRAW A PATTERN ON EACH HALF.

3. SIDE. FRONT. CUT POTATO AWAY FROM THE PATTERN TO LEAVE A RELIEF DESIGN.

4. FOLD EACH PIECE OF PAPER IN HALF PUNCH 3 EYELET HOLES ALONG THE OPEN EDGE OF EACH CARD

5. CUT RIBBON IN 12 INCH LENGTHS.

POTATO PRINT CARDS

6.

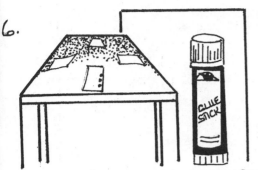

USE GLUE STICK TO SECURE A CARD IN FRONT OF EACH PERSON.

7.

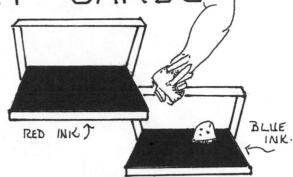

RED INK↑   BLUE INK.

PRESS POTATO DESIGN ON AN INK PAD.

8.

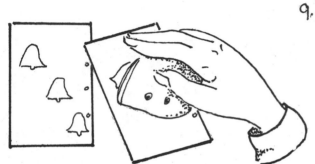

THEN PRESS THE INK COVERED POTATO ON THE PAPER. REPEAT PROCESS MANY TIMES.

PATTERNS FOR CARDS

9.

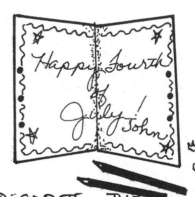

DECORATE THE INSIDE WITH RED AND BLUE FELT PENS. SIGN NAME AND TIE CLOSED. USE RED, WHITE, AND BLUE RIBBONS.

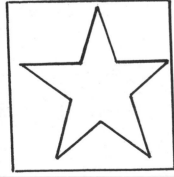

STAR.

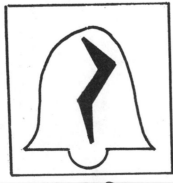

LIBERTY BELL.
(IF DESIRED, GOUGE OUT CRACK IN BELL.)

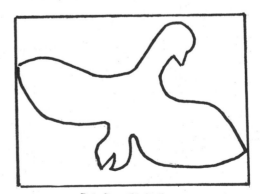

BALD EAGLE.

ENVELOPE FOR CARDS.
APPLY GLUE ON ▨▨▨.
FOLD ON _ _ _ _ _ _.
USE PAPER LARGE ENOUGH
TO HOLD CARDS.

CHAPTER SEVEN

Craft Projects to Sell

TRIVETS

Level of difficulty: *—*****

MATERIALS: Lots of small mosaic tiles or bathroom tiles broken into small bits, craft glue, brush, grout, inexpensive metal hot pads or plastic lazy Susans, damp cloth, bowl and mixing utensil for the grout, water.

APPLICATIONS: These shiny hot pads are handy on any table. If you do not have a metal or plastic backing, just use a smooth board with felt glued on the back.

PREPARATION BEFORE CRAFT SESSION: None.

CRAFT SESSION: Place the tiles on a metal or plastic backing in any pattern or design you like. They should be spaced about ⅛ inch apart. Then glue them in place. When the glue is dry, mix the grout according to the package directions. Fill the cracks with grout and wipe the trivet clean with a damp cloth.

TRIVETS

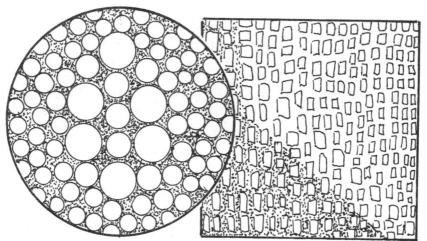

PLASTIC LAZY SUSAN.

METAL HOT PAD.

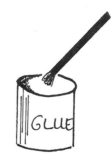

PLACE SMALL MOSAIC TILES ABOUT 1/8 INCH APART IN AN INTERESTING PATTERN. GLUE THEM IN PLACE.

MIX GROUT ACCORDING TO THE DIRECTIONS ON THE PACKAGE.

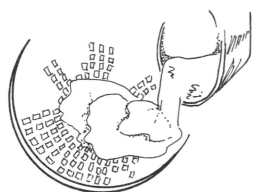

FILL THE CRACKS WITH GROUT.

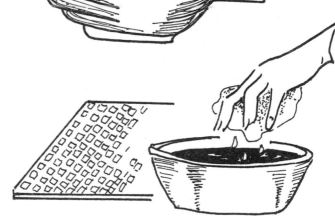

WIPE THE EXCESS GROUT OFF THE TRIVET WITH A DAMP CLOTH.

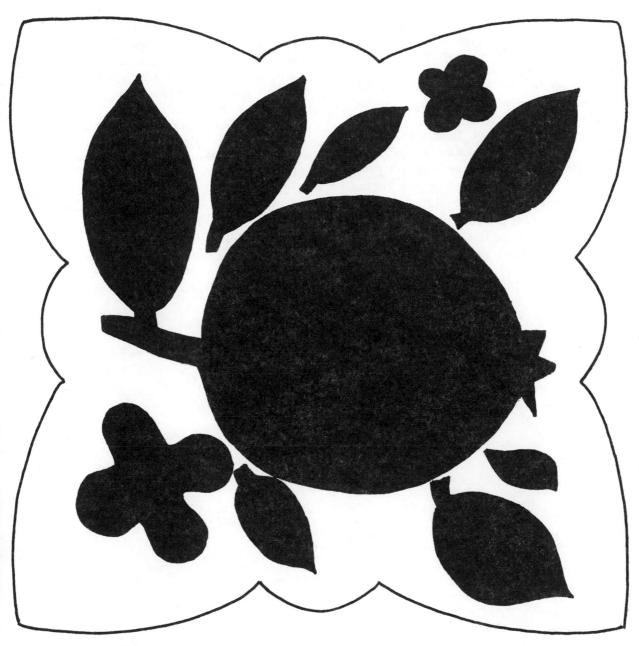

PATTERN FOR TRIVET MADE ON A
WOODEN BOARD. FILL IN THE BLACK
SILHOUETTE WITH TILE BITS OF ONE
COLOR, AND THE BACKGROUND OF ANOTHER.

PIN TINS

Level of difficulty: ***—*****

MATERIALS: Variety of sea shells, empty 3½ ounce tobacco cans with lids (about 4½ inches in diameter), craft glue, brushes, scissors, solid fabric scraps, decorative braid or trim, varnish or craft glaze (optional), pencil.

APPLICATIONS: Sea shells hold a fascination for men, women, and children alike. All will enjoy arranging shells. Try exchanging stories of past trips to beaches. Sell the completed cans as pin tins for dressers. The faint odor of tobacco remains as a pleasant aroma whenever the box is opened.

PREPARATION BEFORE CRAFT SESSION: Wash and dry the tobacco cans. Place a lid on a piece of plain fabric. Trace a circle around the lid and cut it out. Brush the top of the lid with glue and place the circle of fabric on it. Then brush the side of the lid with glue and place braid or decorative trim completely around the circumference of the lid. The lid should now be neatly covered so that its original design does not show.

CRAFT SESSION: Pick out about 24 medium size shells and glue them in place. Keep adding shells until all the crevices are filled and the shells are piled high. For an attractive effect, place some shells upside down or on their side edges. If you like, paint the finished lid with varnish or commercially available craft glaze. Be sure to do this away from patients, as the fumes may be harmful.

PIN TINS

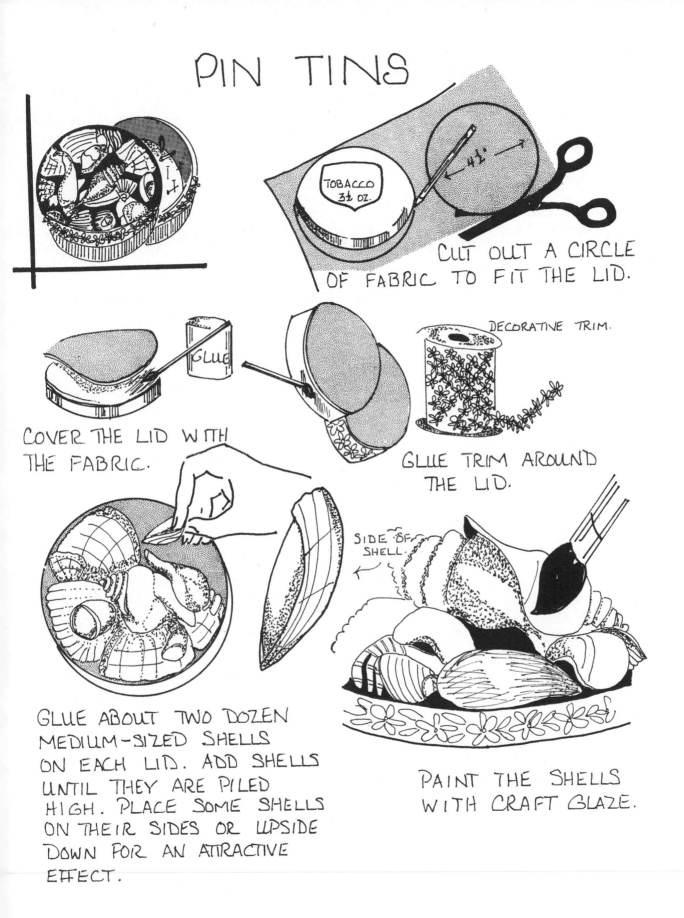

CUT OUT A CIRCLE OF FABRIC TO FIT THE LID.

TOBACCO 3½ OZ.

COVER THE LID WITH THE FABRIC.

GLUE

DECORATIVE TRIM.

GLUE TRIM AROUND THE LID.

GLUE ABOUT TWO DOZEN MEDIUM-SIZED SHELLS ON EACH LID. ADD SHELLS UNTIL THEY ARE PILED HIGH. PLACE SOME SHELLS ON THEIR SIDES OR UPSIDE DOWN FOR AN ATTRACTIVE EFFECT.

SIDE OF SHELL.

PAINT THE SHELLS WITH CRAFT GLAZE.

DECORATIVE BOXES

Level of difficulty: *—*****

MATERIALS: Cigar boxes, craft glue, brush, spring clothespins, scissors, unbleached muslin or felt or paint, dominoes, nuts, bolts, washers.

APPLICATIONS: The clothespin box is attractive enough to become a decorative coffee table box. Try displaying it open and filled with a notepad, pencils, tape, and scissors. Show the domino box filled with cards and scorecards or children's game parts. And show the nuts and bolts box filled with men's accessories.

PREPARATION BEFORE CRAFT SESSION: Cover the cigar boxes with fabric or felt or paint them a solid neutral color. Be sure to cover the insides, too. Remove the springs from the clothespins.

CRAFT SESSION: Choose clothespins, dominoes, or nuts, bolts, and washers to cover a box. Brush glue on the box, a section at a time. Cover the entire box with the decorative objects.

DECORATIVE BOXES

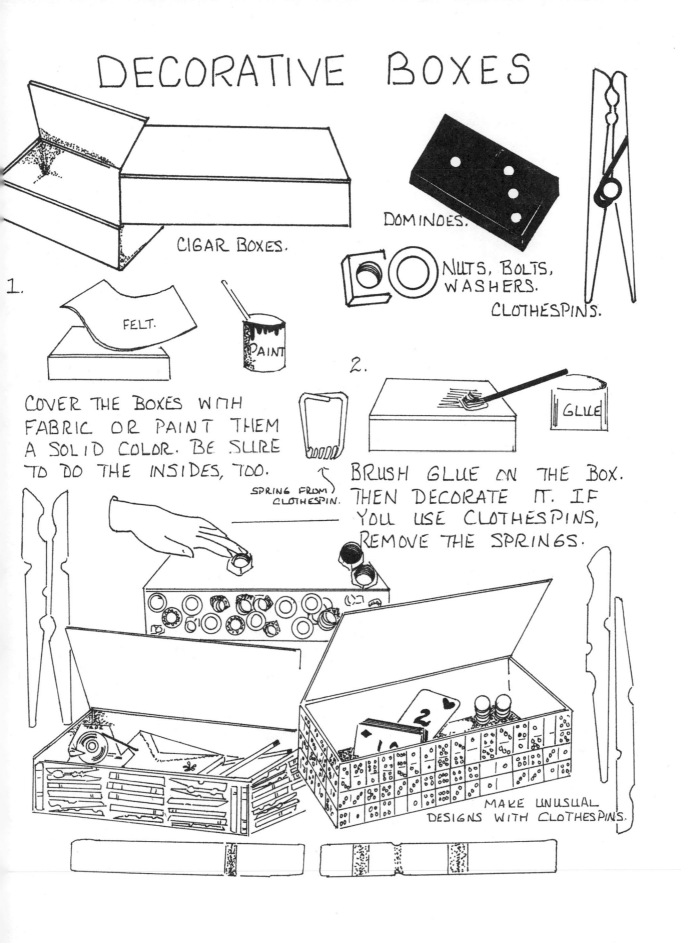

CIGAR BOXES.

DOMINOES.

NUTS, BOLTS, WASHERS.

CLOTHESPINS.

1.

FELT.

PAINT

COVER THE BOXES WITH FABRIC OR PAINT THEM A SOLID COLOR. BE SURE TO DO THE INSIDES, TOO.

SPRING FROM CLOTHESPIN.

2.

GLUE

BRUSH GLUE ON THE BOX. THEN DECORATE IT. IF YOU USE CLOTHESPINS, REMOVE THE SPRINGS.

MAKE UNUSUAL DESIGNS WITH CLOTHESPINS.

WALL HANGINGS

Level of difficulty: ***—*****

MATERIALS: Pink, red, and green felt, scissors, craft glue, brush, heavy cardboard, watermelon seeds, ric rac.

APPLICATIONS: Any kitchen would be brightened by one of these wall hangings. Be creative and make other fruits and vegetables.

PREPARATION BEFORE CRAFT SESSION: Wash and dry some watermelon seeds. Cut cardboard 6 inches by 9 inches. Cut pink felt 6 inches by 9 inches. Follow the patterns in the illustration and cut out the green rind and red watermelon.

CRAFT SESSION: Brush the cardboard with glue. Cover it with pink felt. Glue the green felt on the center of the covered cardboard. Glue the red felt on the center of the green felt. Glue watermelon seeds on the red felt. Trim the wall hanging with ric rac placed about ½ inch from the borders.

WALL HANGINGS

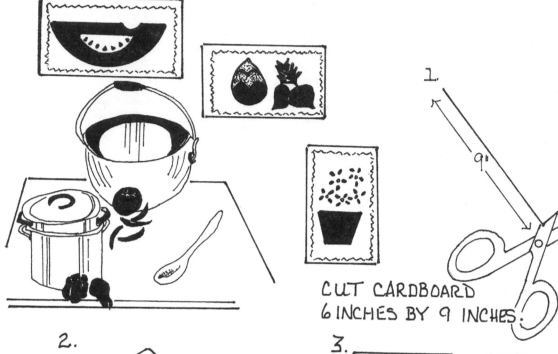

1.
CUT CARDBOARD
6 INCHES BY 9 INCHES.

2.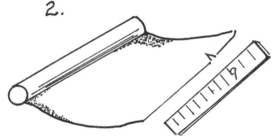

CUT PINK FELT 6 INCHES
BY 9 INCHES.

3. FOLLOW THE
PATTERNS AND CUT OUT
A GREEN FELT RIND AND
A RED FELT WATERMELON.

4.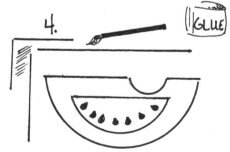

GLUE THE FELT PIECES
ON THE CARDBOARD. ADD
WATERMELON SEEDS.

5.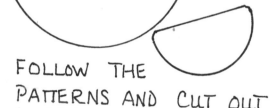

ADD RIC RAC
TRIM ½ INCH FROM
THE BORDERS.

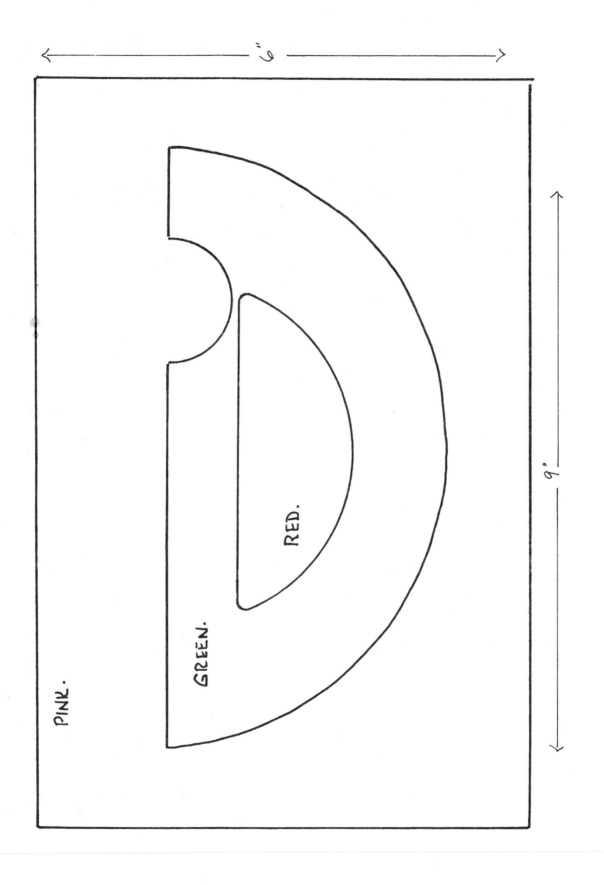

6"

9"

PINK.

GREEN.

RED.

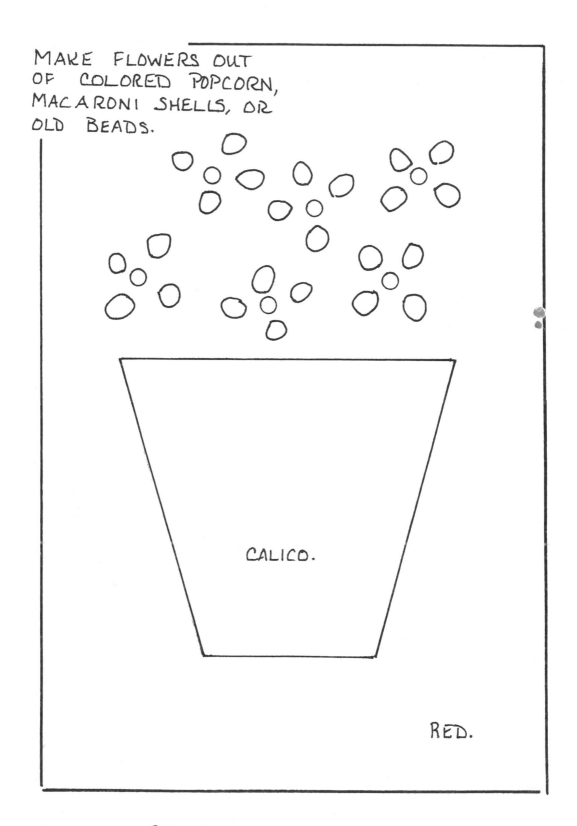

MAKE FLOWERS OUT OF COLORED POPCORN, MACARONI SHELLS, OR OLD BEADS.

CALICO.

RED.

PATTERN FOR WALL HANGINGS.

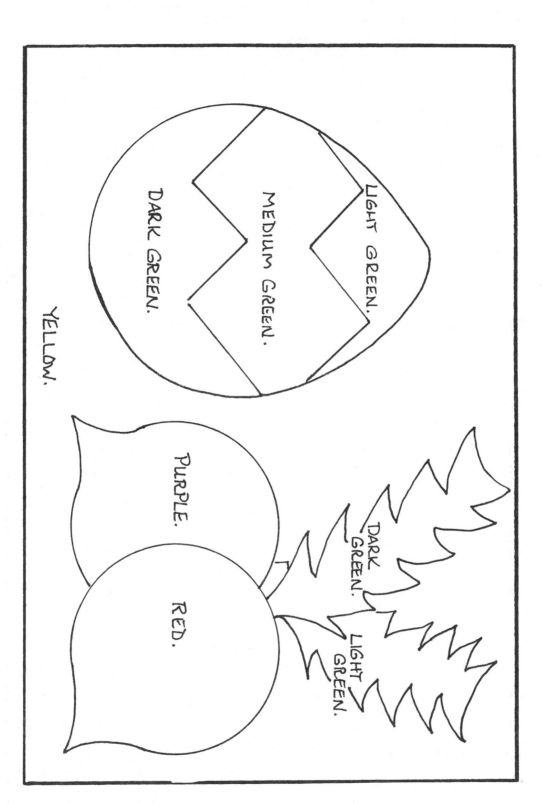

PATTERN FOR WALL HANGINGS.

YELLOW.

DARK GREEN.

MEDIUM GREEN.

LIGHT GREEN.

PURPLE.

RED.

DARK GREEN.

LIGHT GREEN.

STRAWBERRIES

Level of difficulty: *****

MATERIALS: Walnuts, green felt, scissors, small screw eyes, black felt marking pens, gold metallic cord, empty plastic produce baskets, tissue paper, red water-base paint, string, coat hangers, newspapers.

APPLICATIONS: Summer is a good time to make these pretty berry necklaces. If you have a free source for walnuts, make lots of strawberries and arrange them in a basket to sell as table decorations. You may even want to cover the basket with cellophane and tie a pretty bow around it.

PREPARATION BEFORE CRAFT SESSION: Carefully insert a screw eye in one end of each walnut. Cut out one large and one small leaf for each walnut out of green felt.

CRAFT SESSION: Attach one end of a piece of string to a coat hanger. Run the other end of the string through several screw eyes on the walnuts. Then attach this end to the coat hanger. Now dip the walnuts in the red paint and hang them over newspaper to dry. Each individual walnut can be painted with a brush or cotton swab, but hands do get messy. When the nuts are dry, cut the string and remove and save the screw eyes. Place the small leaf on top of the large leaf. Attach the leaves to the walnut by screwing a screw eye through the centers of the leaves at one end of the nut. Then using a black marking pen, make dots all over the painted nut. Run a long piece of gold cord through the screw eye and tie a knot. Make some to fit adults and some to fit children. Display them nicely on a piece of tissue in an empty plastic produce basket.

STRAWBERRIES

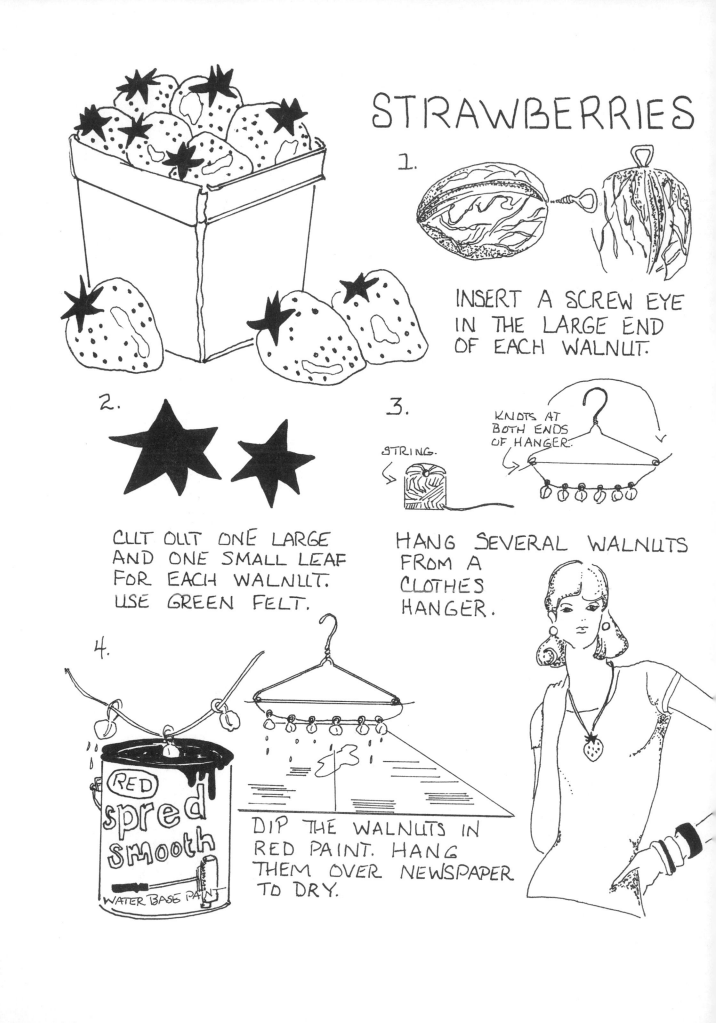

1. INSERT A SCREW EYE IN THE LARGE END OF EACH WALNUT.

2. CUT OUT ONE LARGE AND ONE SMALL LEAF FOR EACH WALNUT. USE GREEN FELT.

3. HANG SEVERAL WALNUTS FROM A CLOTHES HANGER.

STRING.

KNOTS AT BOTH ENDS OF HANGER.

4. RED spred smooth WATER BASE PAINT

DIP THE WALNUTS IN RED PAINT. HANG THEM OVER NEWSPAPER TO DRY.

STRAWBERRIES

5.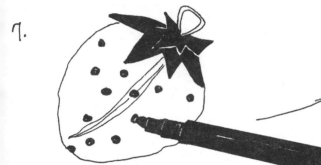

CUT THE STRING. REMOVE AND SAVE THE SCREWEYES.

6.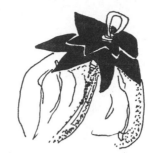

PLACE THE SMALL LEAF ON TOP OF THE LARGE LEAF. ATTACH IT TO THE RED WALNUT WITH A SCREWEYE.

7.

USE A BLACK FELT PEN TO MAKE DOTS ALL OVER THE PAINTED NUT.

8.

TIE A LONG GOLD CORD THROUGH THE SCREWEYE TO MAKE A NECKLACE.

9.

DISPLAY THE NECKLACES ON TISSUE IN EMPTY PLASTIC PRODUCE BASKETS. OR MAKE LOTS OF BERRIES FOR A TABLE DECORATION.

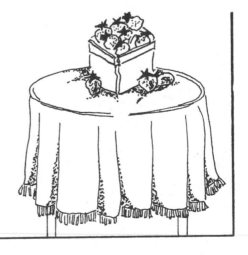

CHRISTMAS ANGELS

Level of difficulty: ****—*****

MATERIALS: Spring clothespins, fabric scraps, net, glitter, craft glue, brush, pop-tops, felt marking pens, pinking shears, scissors, metallic thread, empty margarine tubs, newspaper.

APPLICATIONS: These little angels are practically costless to make and priceless in appeal. Make dozens and cover a tree with them. They will sell themselves.

PREPARATION BEFORE CRAFT SESSION: Follow the pattern in the illustration and using a pinking shears, cut out skirts. Cut out strips of net 12 inches by 6 inches. Cut pieces of metallic thread 12-inches long. Put glitter in one margarine tub and glue in another.

CRAFT SESSION: Draw a face, hair, collar, and hands on the clothespin. You may want to do this on both sides of the clothespin. Dip the 12-inch sides of the net into glue and then into glitter. Shake the net over newspaper to remove the excess glitter. Choose a skirt for the bottom of the clothespin. Secure it with glue. Do this by brushing glue on the clothespin. You may want to dress both sides of the angel. Make a fan out of the net or gather it together in the center and insert it under the spring of the clothespin. Now fan out the wings. Put a loop of thread through the top of the clothespin. Finally, put a pop-top through the angel's head and bend it forward to create a halo. The spring will hold the halo in place. Insert two pop-tops back to back if you are dressing both sides of the angel.

CHRISTMAS ANGELS

1.

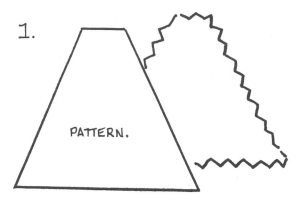

PATTERN.

USING A PINKING SHEARS, FOLLOW THE PATTERN TO CUT OUT SKIRTS.

2.

6"

← 12" →

CUT OUT PIECES OF NET 6 INCHES BY 12 INCHES.

3.

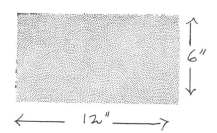

SPRING.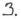

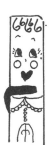 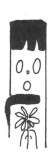

USE FELT PENS TO DRAW FACES, HANDS, COLLARS, AND HAIR ON CLOTHESPINS.

4.

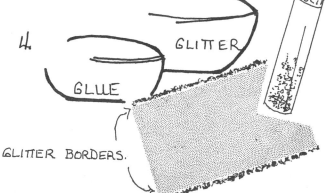

GLITTER

GLUE

GLITTER BORDERS.

DIP THE 12 INCH EDGES OF THE NET INTO GLUE AND THEN INTO GLITTER.

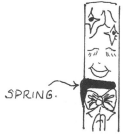

CHRISTMAS ANGELS

5.

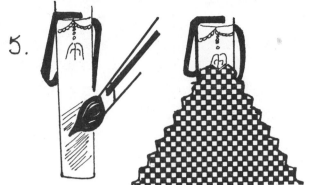

BRUSH GLUE ON THE BOTTOM
OF A CLOTHESPIN AND
ATTACH A SKIRT.

6.

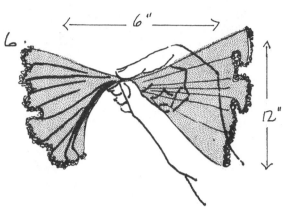

6"

12"

GATHER THE NET
IN THE CENTER.

7.

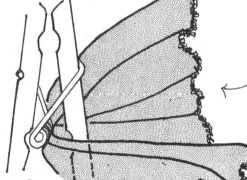

SIDE
VIEWS.

INSERT THE GATHERED
NET UNDER THE SPRING
OF THE CLOTHESPIN.

8.

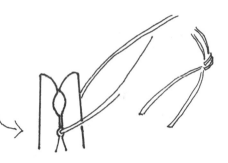

TIE A 12 INCH LOOP OF
METALLIC THREAD THROUGH
THE TOP OF THE CLOTHESPIN.

9.

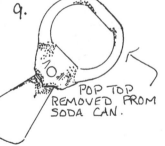

POP TOP
REMOVED FROM
SODA CAN.

PUT A POP TOP THROUGH
THE TOP OF THE ANGEL'S
HEAD. BEND IT FORWARD
TO CREATE A HALO.

10.

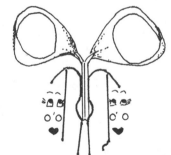

FOR EXTRA ATTRACTIVENESS,
DECORATE BOTH SIDES OF
THE ANGEL. ONE PAIR OF
WINGS IS ENOUGH.

WHEAT HOLDERS

Level of difficulty: ****–*****

MATERIALS: One cup salt, two cups flour, one cup water, putty or kitchen knife, decorative twine or yarn, rolling pin, cookie sheet, cooking oil, varnish or craft glaze, brush, wheat or dried weeds or straw flowers, oven.

APPLICATIONS: These dainty wall vases add a nice flavor of nature to any room. A grouping of several vases is especially appealing. If you have a gift shop, hang some on the wall for an attractive display.

PREPARATION BEFORE CRAFT SESSION: Prepare dough by combing flour and salt in a bowl and mixing well. Add water, a little at a time, mixing as you pour to form a ball. Knead seven to ten minutes until dough is smooth and firm. Oil the cookie sheet.

CRAFT SESSION: Use a rolling pin to roll out dough about ⅜ inch thick. Cut an oval out about 5 inches long by 2½ inches wide. It does not have to be symmetrical. Then cut out a rectangle of dough about 2½ inches wide by 3½ inches long. Lay one finger over the oval as shown in the illustration. Cover that finger with the rectangle of dough. Using the other hand, press the side edges of the rectangle onto the oval. Be certain to moisten all connecting surfaces so that they will bond. Leave the top open. Remove the finger by sliding the hand downward. Then connect the bottom section. Make a small hole in the center of the top of the holder. Bake the completed holder at 325° for 1 hour and 30 minutes or until hard. Let it cool and then coat with varnish or craft glaze. Be sure to do this away from patients, as the fumes may be harmful. Tie a pretty loop through the hole and insert several pieces of wheat or flowers.

WHEAT HOLDERS

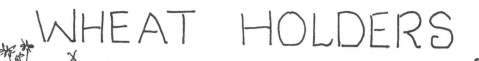

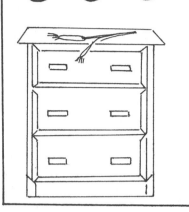

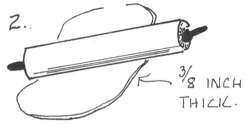

1.

PREPARE DOUGH BY MIXING 1 CUP OF SALT, 2 CUPS OF FLOUR, AND ONE CUP OF WATER. KNEAD THE DOUGH 7 TO 10 MINUTES UNTIL IT IS SMOOTH AND FIRM.

2.

3/8 INCH THICK.

USE A ROLLING PIN TO ROLL THE DOUGH.

3.

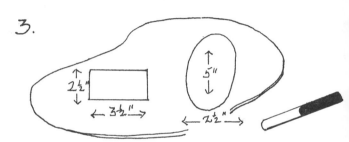

2½"

5"

3½"

2½"

CUT AN OVAL AND A RECTANGLE OUT OF DOUGH.

4.

LAY ONE FINGER OVER THE OVAL.

5.

COVER THAT FINGER WITH THE RECTANGLE OF DOUGH.

WHEAT HOLDERS

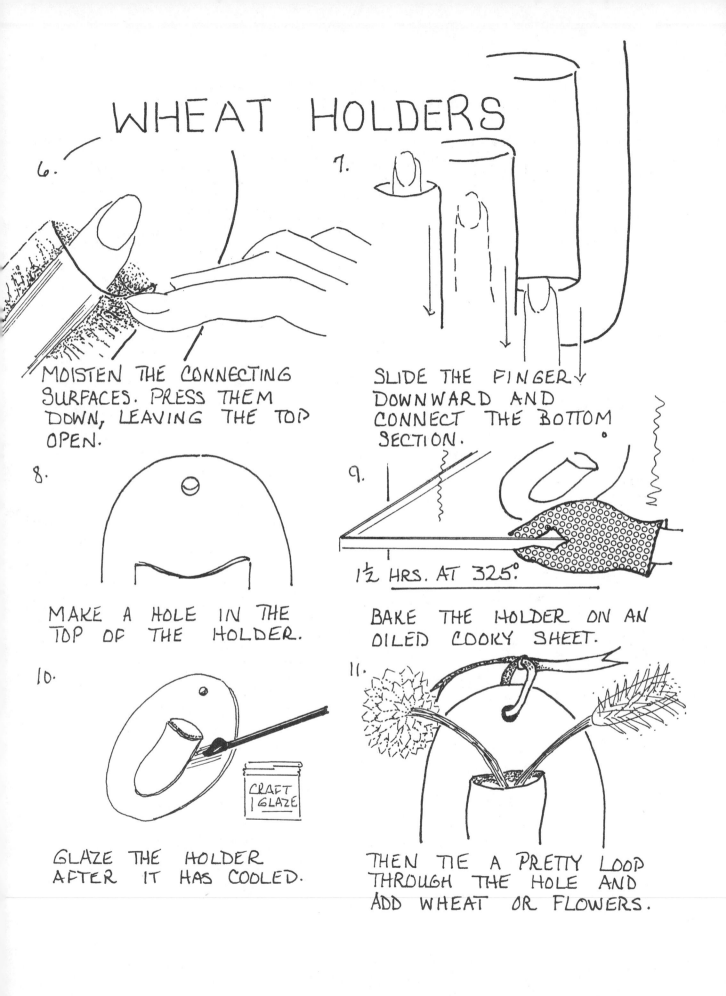

6. MOISTEN THE CONNECTING SURFACES. PRESS THEM DOWN, LEAVING THE TOP OPEN.

7. SLIDE THE FINGER DOWNWARD AND CONNECT THE BOTTOM SECTION.

8. MAKE A HOLE IN THE TOP OF THE HOLDER.

9. 1½ HRS. AT 325°. BAKE THE HOLDER ON AN OILED COOKY SHEET.

10. CRAFT GLAZE. GLAZE THE HOLDER AFTER IT HAS COOLED.

11. THEN TIE A PRETTY LOOP THROUGH THE HOLE AND ADD WHEAT OR FLOWERS.

DECORATED THUMBTACKS

Level of difficulty: ⁎ ⁎ ⁎ ⁎ ⁎

MATERIALS: Thumbtacks (red, yellow, white), permanent black marking pen, plastic wrap and cellophane tape.

APPLICATIONS: Neatly done, these tacks make clever, inexpensive gifts that everyone can use for bulletin boards, offices, kitchens, workshops, or stocking stuffers.

PREPARATION BEFORE CRAFT SESSION: None.

CRAFT SESSION: Decorate the red tacks as apples and ladybugs, the yellow tacks as happy faces, and the white tacks as daisies. Be very careful that the ink does not get on clothing. Using the plastic wrap and tape, rewrap the tacks. Put them onto clean corrogated board if necessary.

DECORATED THUMBTACKS

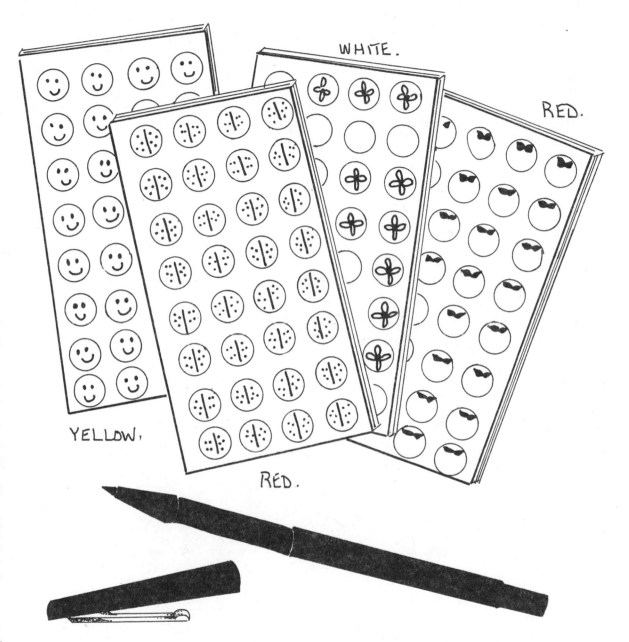

WHITE.

RED.

YELLOW.

RED.

USE A PERMANENT BLACK FELT TIP MARKING PEN. DECORATE YELLOW TACKS AS HAPPY FACES, WHITE TACKS AS DAISIES, AND RED TACKS AS LADYBUGS AND APPLES.

Level of difficulty: **

MATERIALS: Wooden ice cream spoons, felt, felt marking pens, glue, scissors.

APPLICATIONS: Package the decorations in half dozen groups, and display them cleverly. Use imagination to make soldiers, patriots, cowboys, Santas, etc.

PREPARATION BEFORE CRAFT SESSION: Using felt pens, draw faces on the spoons. Precut the felt

CLOWN CUPCAKE DECORATIONS

clothing for the decorations. Assemble the necessary felt pieces and spoons in front of each person. Leave some spoons without faces for those who like to draw.

CRAFT SESSION: Let those who like to draw design their own faces with felt pens. Then have each person glue the felt clothing onto each spoon. Be careful to leave one half of the spoon empty to be inserted into a cupcake.

CUPCAKE DECORATIONS

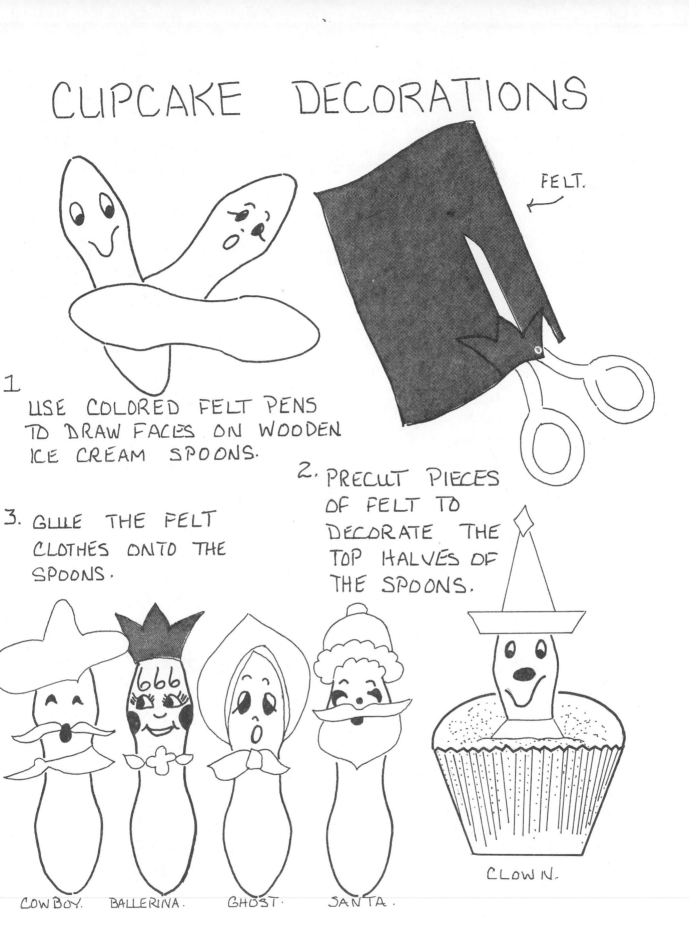

FELT.

1 USE COLORED FELT PENS TO DRAW FACES ON WOODEN ICE CREAM SPOONS.

2. PRECUT PIECES OF FELT TO DECORATE THE TOP HALVES OF THE SPOONS.

3. GLUE THE FELT CLOTHES ONTO THE SPOONS.

COWBOY.   BALLERINA.   GHOST.   SANTA.

CLOWN.

NOTECLIPS

Level of difficulty: *—****

MATERIALS: Spring clothespins, cardboard, felt, colored pipe cleaners, felt marking pens, glue, scissors (ric rac, optional).

APPLICATIONS: These colorful noteclips are clever gifts to sell for any desk or kitchen counter. Clothespins are also useful to keep plastic bags or bread bags tightly closed but easily opened, to attach notes or gasoline receipts to automobile sun visors, and to secure diaper pails bags on car trips.

PREPARATION BEFORE CRAFT SESSION: Cut cardboard and felt the same sizes from patterns, one cardboard and felt pattern for each butterfly and two cardboard and felt patterns for each apple. Cut out dozens of tiny pieces of varied colored felt to decorate the butterflies.

CRAFT SESSION: For the butterfly, draw a happy face with felt pens on the closed end of the clothespin. Then glue the felt to the cardboard and decorate these wings with bits of colored felt and ric rac. Help each person spring the clothespin to slip in the wings and a pipe cleaner for antennae. To make an apple noteclip, glue red felt to the cardboard pattern. Also glue a bit of green pipe cleaner to the back of the cardboard and protruding above the apple to provide a stem. Then glue a felt covered pattern to each side of the clothespin.

NOTECLIPS

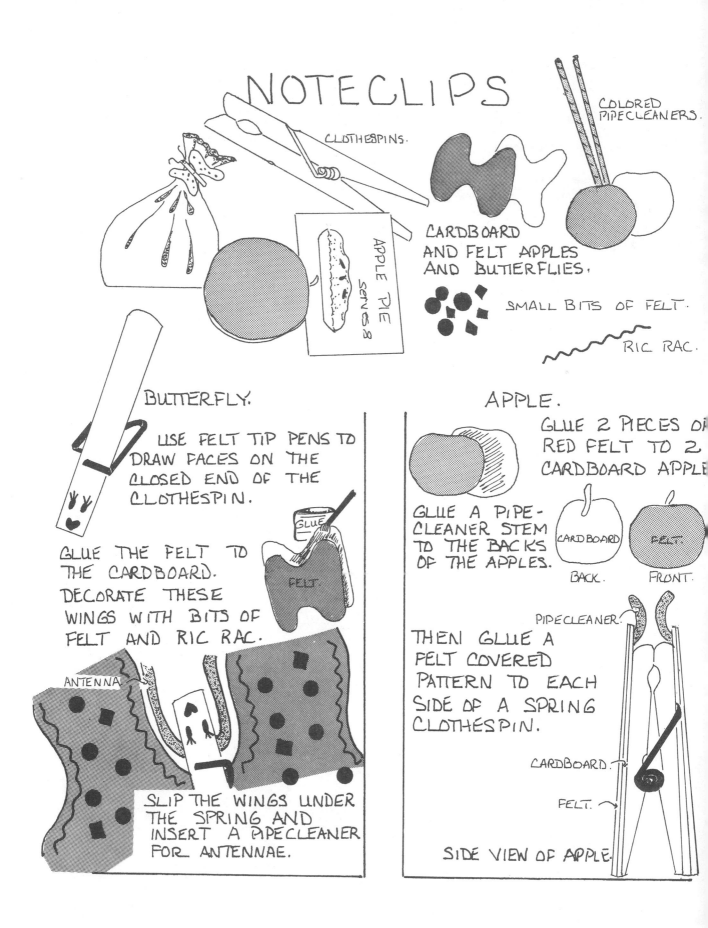

CLOTHESPINS.

COLORED PIPECLEANERS.

CARDBOARD AND FELT APPLES AND BUTTERFLIES.

SMALL BITS OF FELT.

RIC RAC.

APPLE PIE serves 8

BUTTERFLY.

USE FELT TIP PENS TO DRAW FACES ON THE CLOSED END OF THE CLOTHESPIN.

GLUE THE FELT TO THE CARDBOARD. DECORATE THESE WINGS WITH BITS OF FELT AND RIC RAC.

GLUE
FELT.

ANTENNA

SLIP THE WINGS UNDER THE SPRING AND INSERT A PIPECLEANER FOR ANTENNAE.

APPLE.

GLUE 2 PIECES OF RED FELT TO 2 CARDBOARD APPLES

GLUE A PIPE-CLEANER STEM TO THE BACKS OF THE APPLES.

CARDBOARD   FELT

BACK.   FRONT.

PIPECLEANER.

THEN GLUE A FELT COVERED PATTERN TO EACH SIDE OF A SPRING CLOTHESPIN.

CARDBOARD.

FELT.

SIDE VIEW OF APPLE.

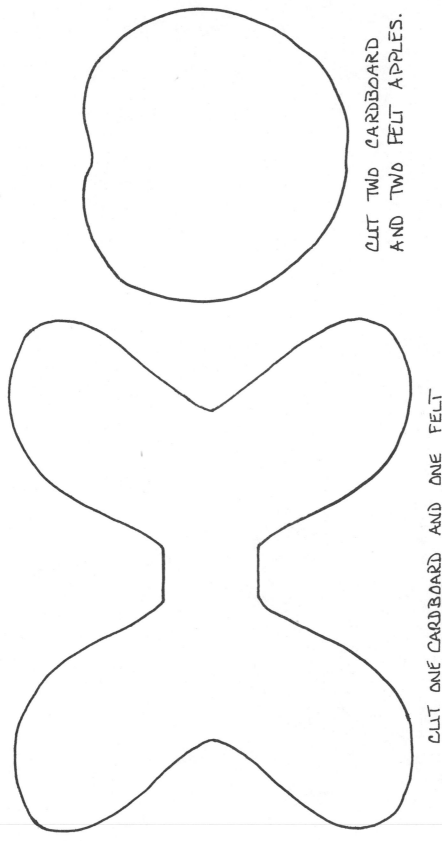

PATTERNS FOR NOTECLIPS

CUT TWO CARDBOARD AND TWO FELT APPLES.

CUT ONE CARDBOARD AND ONE FELT BUTTERFLY.

Bibliography

Bonner, Charles D.: *Medical Care and Rehabilitation of the Aged and Chronically Ill.* Boston, Little, 1974.

Brocklehurst, J. C.: *Textbook of Geriatrics Medicine and Gerontology.* Edinburgh, Churchill Livingstone, 1973.

Brook, Peter; Degun, Gian; and Mather, Marcia: Reality Orientation, A Therapy for Psychogeriatric Patients: A Controlled Study. *Br J Psychiatry, 127:* 42-5, 1975.

Busse, Ewald W. and Pfiffer, Eric: *Mental Illness in Later Life.* Washington, D. C., American Psychiatric Association, 1973.

Butler, Robert N.: *Why Survive? Being Old in America.* New York, Har-Row, 1975.

Coleman, James C.: *Abnormal Psychology and Modern Life.* Glenview, Scott Foresman, 1964.

Cowdry, E. V. and Steinberg, Franz U.: *The Care of the Geriatric Patient.* Saint Louis, Mosby, 1971.

Cruickshank, William M.: *Psychology of Exceptional Children and Youth.* Englewood Cliffs, P-H, 1963.

Ferguson, Elizabeth A.: *Social Work.* Philadelphia, Lippincott, 1963.

Gould, Elaine and Gould, Loren: *Crafts for the Elderly.* Springfield, Thomas, 1971.

Harris, Jay and Joseph, Cliff: *Murals of the Mind.* New York, Intl Univs Pr, 1973.

Isaacs, Bernard: *An Introduction to Geriatrics.* Baltimore, Williams and Wilkins, 1965.

Jaeger, Dorothea and Simmons, Leo W.: *The Aged Ill.* New York, Appleton, 1970.

Kessler, Henry H.: *Disability—Determination and Evaluation.* Philadelphia, Lea and Febiger, 1970.

Kimmel, Douglas C.: *Adulthood and Aging.* New York, Wiley, 1974.

Nagi, Saad Z.: *Disability and Rehabilitation.* Ohio St U Pr, 1969.

Quilitch, H. Robert: Purposeful Activity Increased on a Geriatrics Ward Through Programmed Recreation. *Journal of the American Geriatrics Society, Vol. XXII,* 5:226-29, 1974.

Rossman, Isadore: *Clinical Geriatrics.* Philadelphia, Lippincott, 1971.

Simpson, George: *People in Families.* New York, Crowell Collier, 1960.

Walters, Barbara: *How to Talk With Practically Anybody About Practically Anything.* Garden City, Doubleday, 1970.

Willard, Helen S. and Spackman, Clare S.: *Occupational Therapy.* Philadelphia, Lippincott, 1971.

Wolff, Kurt: *The Biological, Sociological and Psychological Aspects of Aging.* Springfield, Thomas, 1959.